# Integrating Digital Tools Into Children's Mental Health Care

## About the Authors

**Deborah J. Jones**, PhD, is the Zachary Smith Distinguished Term Professor and Associate Chair of Psychology and Neuroscience at the University of North Carolina at Chapel Hill. She has had multiple grants from the National Institute of Mental Health to study the role of digital tools in children's mental health and has over 100 publications on related topics. She also teaches a digital mental health course at the university.

**Margaret T. Anton**, PhD, is a senior clinical innovation and research manager at Two Chairs, a behavioral health company using technology and design to improve the process of accessing and receiving quality mental health care. Over the past ten years, she has developed, evaluated, and implemented technology-enabled behavioral interventions in academic, community, and industry settings.

## Advances in Psychotherapy – Evidence-Based Practice



The basic objective of this series is to provide therapists with practical, evidence-based treatment guidance for the most common disorders seen in clinical practice – and to do so in a reader-friendly manner. Each book in the series is both a compact "how-to" reference on a particular disorder for use by professional clinicians in their daily work and an ideal educational resource for students as well as for practice-oriented continuing education.

The most important feature of the books is that they are practical and easy to use: All are structured similarly and all provide a compact and easy-to-follow guide to all aspects that are relevant in real-life practice. Tables, boxed clinical "pearls," marginal notes, and summary boxes assist orientation, while checklists provide tools for use in daily practice.

### Continuing Education Credits

Psychologists and other healthcare providers may earn five continuing education credits for reading the books in the *Advances in Psychotherapy* series and taking a multiple-choice exam. This continuing education program is a partnership of Hogrefe Publishing and the National Register of Health Service Psychologists. Details are available at https://www.hogrefe.com/us/cenatreg

The National Register of Health Service Psychologists is approved by the American Psychological Association to sponsor continuing education for psychologists. The National Register maintains responsibility for this program and its content.

Advances in Psychotherapy – Evidence-Based Practice, Volume 52

# Integrating Digital Tools Into Children's Mental Health Care

**Deborah J. Jones**
University of North Carolina at Chapel Hill, NC

**Margaret T. Anton**
Two Chairs, San Francisco, CA

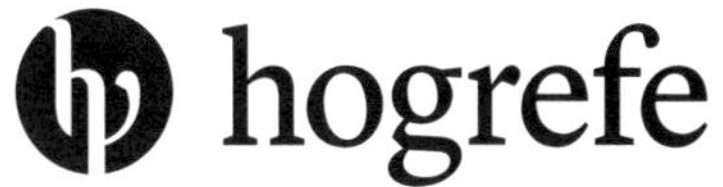

**Library of Congress of Congress Cataloging in Publication** information for the print version of this book is available via the Library of Congress Marc Database under the Library of Congress Control Number 2023943287

**Library and Archives Canada Cataloguing in Publication**

Title: Integrating digital tools into children's mental health care / Deborah J. Jones, University of North Carolina at Chapel Hill, NC ; Margaret T. Anton, Two Chairs, San Francisco, CA.
Names: Jones, Deborah J. (Deborah Jean), 1971- author. | Anton, Margaret T., author.
Series: Advances in psychotherapy--evidence-based practice ; v. 52.
Description: Series statement: Advances in psychotherapy--evidence-based practice ; volume 52 | Includes bibliographical references.
Identifiers: Canadiana (print) 20230504612 | Canadiana (ebook) 20230504604 | ISBN 9780889376014 (softcover) | ISBN 9781613346013 (EPUB) | ISBN 9781616766016 (PDF)
Subjects: LCSH: Mentally ill children—Care—Technological innovations. | LCSH: Child mental health services—Technological innovations.
Classification: LCC RJ499 .J66 2023 | DDC 618.92/8900285—dc23



www.hogrefe.com



PUBLISHING OFFICES

| | |
|---|---|
| USA: | Hogrefe Publishing Corporation, 44 Merrimac St., Suite 207, Newburyport, MA 01950<br>Phone 978 255 3700; E-mail customersupport@hogrefe.com |
| EUROPE: | Hogrefe Publishing GmbH, Merkelstr. 3, 37085 Göttingen, Germany<br>Phone +49 551 99950 0, Fax +49 551 99950 111; E-mail publishing@hogrefe.com |

SALES & DISTRIBUTION

| | |
|---|---|
| USA: | Hogrefe Publishing, Customer Services Department,<br>30 Amberwood Parkway, Ashland, OH 44805<br>Phone 800 228 3749, Fax 419 281 6883; E-mail customersupport@hogrefe.com |
| UK: | Hogrefe Publishing, c/o Marston Book Services Ltd., 160 Eastern Ave.,<br>Milton Park, Abingdon, OX14 4SB<br>Phone +44 1235 465577, Fax +44 1235 465556; E-mail direct.orders@marston.co.uk |
| EUROPE: | Hogrefe Publishing, Merkelstr. 3, 37085 Göttingen, Germany<br>Phone +49 551 99950 0, Fax +49 551 99950 111; E-mail publishing@hogrefe.com |

OTHER OFFICES

| | |
|---|---|
| CANADA: | Hogrefe Publishing Corporation, 82 Laird Drive, East York, Ontario, M4G 3V1 |
| SWITZERLAND: | Hogrefe Publishing, Länggass-Strasse 76, 3012 Bern |



Printed and bound in the USA

ISBN 978-0-88937-601-4 (print) • ISBN 978-1-61676-601-6 (PDF) • ISBN 978-1-61334-601-3 (EPUB)
https://doi.org/10.1027/00601-000

# Dedication

We dedicate this book to the mentors who instilled in us the importance of the link between research and practice and the children and families with whom we have worked in both domains.

# Acknowledgments

We are grateful to the American Psychological Association (APA Division 12) and Hogrefe for producing a book that aims to bridge the research-to-practice gap in children's mental health. We thank our series editor, Jonathan Comer, for allowing us to share our knowledge and experience toward practical guidance for clinicians interested in incorporating digital tools into their practice. Dr. Jones also extends her gratitude to the APA Division 12 Task Force on Digital Mental Health (Jenna Carl, Jon Comer, Brian Doss, Oliver Lindhiem, Adela Timmons, Ken Weingardt). Participation in this group has profoundly enriched my understanding of the nuances inherent in the impact of digital innovation on mental health service delivery and the critical importance of collaboration between industry, academics, practitioners, and policymakers. Finally, both Dr. Anton and Dr. Jones would like to acknowledge the children and families with whom we have worked as our experiences with them helped to shape our interest in digital mental health.

# Contents

# Preface

COVID-19 and associated stay-at-home and social distancing public health guidelines dramatically expedited the use of digital tools in mental health generally, and children's mental health is no exception (see Sullivan et al., 2021; Torous et al., 2022 for reviews). Changes in reimbursement policies for remote services have further paved the way for new service delivery models and options. Although vaccination efforts should ultimately allow for the resumption of in-person services, telemental health and other digital mental health approaches and tools will likely continue to be a part of the children's mental health landscape moving forward.

As such progress unfolds, we are reminded of a quote by Steve Jobs, Apple cofounder, in a 1994 *Rolling Stone* interview: "Technology is nothing. What's important is that you have faith in people, that they're basically good and smart, and if you give them tools, they'll do wonderful things with them" (Goodell, 2011) We use this quote when training therapists, working clinically with children and families, and presenting our research at conferences as it echoes our evaluation of the role of digital tools in children's mental health as well. That is, technology is one tool that clinicians have at their disposal that may help to increase access to, engagement in, and/or outcomes of evidence-based clinical practice. Accordingly, we aim to provide evidence-based and practical clinical information and illustrations along with supporting didactic materials to guide clinician adoption and integration of digital tools in assessment and treatment plans with children and families.

This book is divided into five chapters. Chapter 1 describes the broad range of terminology used in digital mental health. Chapter 2 reviews some leading theoretical approaches that highlight the mechanisms through which it is posited that digital tools can increase access to, engagement in, and outcomes of evidence-based mental health services for children and families. In Chapter 3, we present guidance for therapeutic decision making regarding if, when, and for whom digital tools may be most useful. Chapter 4 presents examples of ways in which digital tools can be incorporated into clinical practice, the efficacy data available for such examples, and common obstacles to successful outcomes. Finally, Chapter 5 presents case examples that describe the incorporation of digital tools into clinical practice. A variety of forms and handouts to guide the use of digital tools and related decision making are presented in the Appendix. One that may be helpful even before you dive into the first chapter on terminology is the Provider Self-Assessment of Technology Comfort and Attitudes handout in Appendix 1. Importantly, there is no scoring system or right or wrong answers to these questions. Rather, we hope that this assessment will encourage you to think about your comfort with and attitudes toward digital mental health and incorporating digital tools into your clinical care with child clients and their families. It may be helpful to revisit the questions as you work your way through each chapter of the book to see if your comfort and attitudes are changing and if so how.

# 1

# Description

## 1.1 Terminology

Digital mental health and the terms used to describe it are evolving quickly much like technology generally. To clarify how we are using the terms for the purposes of this book, we chose to start here with those that we think are most reflective of the broader state of the digital mental health field. As the book continues, we emphasize the specific relevance of digital tools in children's mental health in particular using more of a developmental lens, including theory, assessment and treatment, and case vignettes.

## 1.2 Definition

**Use of digital, mobile, and connected technologies in assessment and treatment**

Digital mental health broadly refers to the use of digital, mobile, and connected technologies to advance assessment and treatment. The range of digital tools available to mental health providers continues to rapidly evolve. These include the use of electronic records, which is now standard in children's mental health, but also a broader range of digital tools including examples highlighted in Box 1 and discussed in this chapter and throughout this volume. Our aim with this book is to maintain our focus on the promise of digital mental health, while also staying grounded in the evidence base underlying the rationale for this approach.

## 1.3 Telemental Health

Telemental health (or telehealth or teletherapy) generally refers to the use of video and audio data to facilitate therapist-led, synchronous (i.e., real-time) mental health care. A mass transition to telemental health was necessary for providers and clients at the start of the COVID-19 pandemic and associated stay-at-home and social distancing public health mandates. Accordingly, whereas telemental health was not a dominant mode of mental health care delivery prior to the COVID-19 pandemic, it has now entered the clinical mainstream (Comer, 2021). Generally, telemental health requires the provider and client both have a device (e.g., laptop computer, tablet, phone) with audio and/or video-display functionality, a web camera, and nonpublic facing, Health Insurance Privacy and Portability Act (HIPAA)-compliant videoconferencing software (e.g., Doxy.me, Vidyo).

### 1.3.1 Nonpublic Facing Video Communication

**Nonpublic facing video communication requiring logins and passwords is one HIPAA criterion**

There are generally two broad categories of videoconferencing software available to consumers – public and nonpublic facing. Public facing video communication software essentially refers to a software that allows video communication that is open or accessible to the public (e.g., Facebook Live, TikTok, Twitch) that generally precludes the possibility for confidentiality, privacy, or data security necessary for digital mental health. In contrast, nonpublic facing video communication uses end-to-end encryption or encoding of data (e.g., audio, video, text) that allows only the client (i.e., child, parent) and the mental health service provider to hear, see, or read the audio, video, or text that is being exchanged and vice versa. Nonpublic facing platforms also generally require individual user accounts (e.g., logins, passwords) to limit and verify users, as well settings relevant to privacy and security (e.g., choice to record, mute, or turn off the video or audio). Nonpublic facing video communication software (e.g., Zoom for Healthcare, Doxy.me, Thera-Link) is one criterion to meet current HIPAA standards, although there are others as well which are listed in Box 2 and described next in further detail.

### 1.3.2 HIPAA Compliance

What makes a telemental health (or any other digital) platform HIPAA compliant generally relates to how digital data (e.g., voice, audio, text) are transferred and stored (e.g., encryption). HIPAA standards are generally the responsibility of both the videoconferencing vendor and the clinician via a business associate agreement (BAA). The BAA is typically embedded within the terms of software use and makes explicit within those terms of use and accountability what happens should a HIPAA breach occur. Many nonpublic facing videoconferencing software platforms have BAAs (e.g., Zoom for Healthcare, Doxy.me, Thera-Link). Although there was a grace period extended at the start of the COVID-19 pandemic that emphasized the mental health providers' good faith efforts to provide HIPAA-compliant remote-service delivery, ongoing awareness and education regarding the appropriateness of various options is essential. For example, Apple's Facetime (and iCloud) meet many data privacy and security standards relevant to HIPAA compliance; however, their terms of use state that they do not constitute a BAA, should not be used for business that requires HIPAA compliance, and that they will not accept responsibility if a HIPAA or Health Information Technology for Economic and Clinical Health (HITECH) Act breach occurs. To ensure HIPAA compliance in one's telemental health practice, it is always recommended that legal counsel first review the selected telemental health platform and associated BAA.

### 1.3.3 HITECH Act

**Digital mental health tools must comply with HIPAA and HITECH**

The HITECH Act, which was signed into law by President Obama, was instituted as part of the American Recovery and Reinvestment Act of 2009 as a part of a broader economic stimulus bill. HITECH was enacted to promote the implementation and use of electronic health records with the goal of achieving a more efficient, integrated, and cost-effective health care system. Embedded within HITECH (Subtitle D) is the mandate for privacy and security associated with the electronic transmission of health information, including enforcement of HIPAA rules and consequences for HIPAA breaches and violations. Although focused initially on electronic health records, companies that market and support videoconferencing and other mobile mental health interventions typically refer to both HIPAA and HITECH in their terms of use.

### 1.3.4 Reimbursement

Prior to the COVID-19 pandemic, most payers, including Medicaid and Medicare, did not reimburse telemental health services provided in patients' homes and only five states offered telehealth parity for mental health conditions. As a result, fewer than 10% of the US population had used telehealth for a clinical encounter prior to the COVID-19 pandemic (Warren & Smalley, 2020). When a public health emergency was declared, it included emergency orders that rapidly increased access to and reimbursement for telemental health services. The uptake of telehealth services both for clinicians and their clients skyrocketed and thrust us into an era where most providers became familiar with this delivery method and most clients had access to these services if they preferred. Now, nearly 40% of the US population has used telehealth, and there is a desire from both providers and clients to continue to have telehealth options after the pandemic (American Psychiatric Association, 2021). Public guidance will likely continue to adapt and change over time, including if and how telemental health and other digital interventions are covered by insurance. Providers should stay up to date through organizations such as the American Psychological Association (APA) or other professional associations and agencies, as well as state licensing boards and relevant insurance panels.

## 1.4 Mobile (Mental) Health

The World Health Organization (WHO) defines mobile health (also known as mHealth) broadly "as the use of mobile wireless technologies for public health" (Executive Board, 2017). Telemental health can also be included within mobile mental health, given that videoconferencing software, for example, can be used on a clinician's or family's mobile phone or tablet. Providers may also use mobile technologies to augment or supplement face-to-face treatment, including between-session video coaching calls (e.g., check-in, problem-solving, promoting skill generalizability) and the assignment of mental health software applications (apps) (Jones et al., 2014, 2021; Parent et al., 2022). As such, in the next section we provide an overview of some of the most common digital tools and approaches; however, we do not want to falsely suggest that these are all necessarily distinct. Rather, a clinician providing either in-person or telemental health services may use multiple additional tools and approaches throughout their care of a client.

## 1.5 Mental Health Apps

An app is a software program that uses the operating system on the device on which it is loaded to allow the user to do various tasks or activities. Apps for desktop or laptop computers are sometimes called desktop applications, whereas those for smartphones, tablets, and wearables (e.g., smart watches), for example, are called mobile apps. With 85% of Americans now owning a smartphone (Pew Research Center, 2019) and 130 billion app downloads in 2020, the number of mobile apps for mental health are rapidly proliferating. Furthermore, current data suggest that the move to "cut-the-cord" on landlines is equally if not more prevalent in low-income homes, which are also more likely to rely on mobile phones as their primary if not only device. Mental health apps offer tremendous potential to decrease mental health care disparities and can be used by clinicians to strengthen and extend the reach of services.

**Most mental health apps have not been evaluated, making clinician review important**

The ubiquity of mobile devices also opens the door for a range of other digital tools that are being increasingly democratized, including virtual reality (i.e., user immersed in technology), augmented reality (i.e., technology integrated into real world of user), and video games, each of which are defined in detail in subsequent sections in this chapter. That said, only 3–4% of the estimated 10,000–20,000 mobile mental health apps available to consumers are considered evidence based, making it critical for clinicians to investigate and evaluate efficacy data before incorporating these apps into treatment (Bry et al., 2018; Larsen et al., 2019; Lecomte et al., 2020). OneMind PsyberGuide attempts to provide consumers with information on currently available mobile mental health apps as well as available data and expert reviews; however, relatively few of the included apps focus on children's mental health (see Appendix 8).

To help you consider how to select and incorporate a mobile app into clinical work with your clients, we encourage you to see the handout in Appendix 2: Exploring and Identifying a Digital Tool to Integrate Into Child Mental Health Care. As the instructions highlight, we focus on mobile apps as an example of a digital tool, so it may be a useful exercise to consider here or at the end of this chapter. You may also revisit these prompts as you consider incorporating other digital tools into your practice.

## 1.6 Digital Therapeutics

Digital therapeutics are a category of digital mental health tools defined as evidence-based therapeutic interventions driven by software programs that aim to prevent, manage, or treat physical, mental, or behavioral conditions (Digital Therapeutics Alliance, 2020). Digital therapeutics are distinguished from the broader category of consumer mental health and wellness apps because they are classified as "Software as a Medical Device" by the International Medical Device Regulators Forum (IMDRF, 2014), which requires review and oversight. In the United States, for example, the FDA has designated digital therapeutics for mental and behavioral health as "prescription-only" tools, which has significant implications for if, how, and by whom they can be used (see Carl et al., 2020, 2022; Torous et al., 2022 for reviews). On one hand, such regulation has the potential to provide improved quality assurance and legitimize digital approaches to treatment and, in turn, inform and guide providers in the standard of care digital tools for their practice. At the same time, only the limited number of mental health providers with "prescription privileges" can prescribe these tools to their clients (Doss et al., 2021). In addition, there is much discussion about whether the FDA is using the most valid criteria (e.g., symptom reduction, quality of life) to evaluate the efficacy of digital therapeutics (Carl et al., 2020, 2022), in turn making the selection of "evidence-based" digital tools more complicated for providers. Finally, digital therapeutics are largely being cleared as prescribed adjuncts to clinical care or essentially a technology-enhanced treatment; however, stand-alone treatments could also be an option.

## 1.7 Stand-Alone Treatments

Stand-alone digital mental health tools are generally considered those which individuals, in our case children and/or their families, can access and use directly. These tools include self-guided programs, as well as those that include a human support or coaching component. Self-guided tools include apps designed to aid in symptom monitoring, provide interactive activities designed to enhance skills, and provide symptom relief in the moment (e.g., distress tolerance and mindfulness activities). Stand-alone programs that include human support or coaching are designed to accomplish the same things as self-guided programs, but also offer support designed to enhance engagement, guide use, and reinforce skill use and practice. Support can range from chatbot support to asynchronous in-app messaging to weekly phone/video-based check-ins with coaches. Coaches are generally paraprofessionals trained in basic behavior change principles and motivational intervention. Although there is some overlap between coaching and traditional clinical care, the role of coaches is more limited and not meant to replace more intensive one-on-one treatment. For example, in one of the most prevalent and evidence-based coaching models, known as supportive accountability, coaching is thought to enhance engagement by holding the participant accountable to the coach who is seen as trustworthy, helpful, and having expertise. Accountability is established through setting up clear expectations collaboratively with the participant and having reciprocity in the relationship, one in which the participants feel supported and understand the benefit of ongoing engagement (Mohr et al., 2011). While both self-guided and coached stand-alone interventions have been shown to be effective, research consistently demonstrates that coaching improves app/program engagement and leads to improved clinical outcomes.

**Clinical Pearl**

When Clinicians May Recommend Stand-Alone Treatment

Clinicians may have some reluctance about stand-alone digital tools, given that they may be seen as a replacement for in-person services. Yet, the reach and impact of evidence-based mental health care has been challenged by the inaccessibility and limited acceptability of the traditional model of clinic-based service delivery, and most (50–80%) youth, particularly those outside of urban and university communities of youth, do not receive services (American Psychological Association, 2018, 2021; Comer & Barlow, 2014; Kazdin & Blase, 2011). For example, rural children experience comparable rates of mental health problems as children in other geographic regions; however, they are 20% less likely to receive mental health care than urban and suburban children, a rate that rises to 50% less likely when impairment is moderate (Fehr et al., 2020; Sullivan et al., 2021). Given meta-analytic findings suggesting that digital tools can be effective both as adjuncts or stand-alone treatments (Lindhiem et al., 2015), they hold promise to broaden the reach and impact of evidence-based mental health care including to the most vulnerable and underserved by our traditional clinic-based mental health care system. Indeed, decisions regarding if and who may benefit from using digital tools as an enhancement or a replacement for in-person treatment may depend on accessibility (i.e., stand-alone intervention is the only treatment option), as well as level of risk (e.g., higher level of risk may benefit most from in-person services enhanced with digital tools). As such, providers may consider recommending stand-alone digital mental health tools for children and families in regions traditionally underserved by mental health providers, populations for which stigma is a long-standing and entrenched barrier to care, and/or when problems are perhaps subclinical (i.e., prevention) and/or wait-lists delay in-person care (i.e., gateway to in-person care).

## 1.8 Digital Games

Digital or video games are played by millions. Numerous studies have demonstrated the potentially harmful effects of playing video games in children, including increased risk for aggression, addiction, and depression in some children (Ferrari et al., 2020). In turn, WHO has now identified the new classification of gaming disorder characterized by a pattern of lack or loss of control, precedence over other daily activities, and continuation in spite of negative consequences. Such trends may make clinicians cautious about recommending digital games as an assessment or treatment tool for children and families. That said, the ubiquity of digital games simultaneously highlights the potential to be a convenient, familiar, and thus potentially engaging digital mental health tool as well. To that end, some data exist to suggest that games can help children improve their attention span, develop problem-solving skills, manage emotions, and assist with treatment for a range of disorders (Ferrari et al., 2020).

The Smartphone-Enhanced Child Anxiety Treatment (SmartCAT) is a smartphone app that was developed to augment traditional face-to-face treatment for child anxiety (Pramana et al., 2014). After pilot testing, the developers engaged in a redesign process to add gamification to promote engagement. The SmartCAT tool now includes interactive games and activities designed to reinforce skill knowledge, an in vivo skills coach that prompts the client to use skills when experiencing real-world distress, a challenge to promote home-based exposure practice, and a digital reward system that contains points that can be traded in for trophies and other digital rewards (Pramana et al., 2018). The developers found that the addition of the gamification features boosted engagement in SmartCAT as well as the intervention overall (see also Silk et al., 2020).

## 1.9 Augmented and Virtual Reality

As noted earlier, augmented reality uses technology to overlay sight, sound, touch, or other sensory information onto the user's real-world experience. Common examples of augmented reality wearables available to consumers include smart glasses (e.g., Google Glass, Microsoft HoloLens, Oculus Quest). Research on augmented reality and youth is in the very nascent phase, and only a few small case studies exist to date. One example is a smartglass intervention for youth with autism spectrum disorders called Brain Power System. Brain Power System has several gamified, augmented reality interventions built into the smartglass system, including one called Face Game, designed to increase face gazing. The system overlays cartoon features on faces detected in the individual's visual field to improve and reinforce eye contact. Digital features are removed as the child learns to interact on their own (Liu et al., 2017).

**Virtual reality has been used in both training of providers and treatment of children and families**

Virtual reality or technology allows the opposite, which is to immerse the consumer in a virtual environment. Such technology has been available to consumers for longer than augmented reality and has been at least preliminary tested in the children's mental health literature (see Halldorsson et al., 2021 for a review). Although still largely at its preliminary stages, virtual reality has been tested in the assessment and treatment of children with social skills deficits, including those with autism (e.g., Maskey et al., 2019), as well as social anxiety (e.g., Le & Beidel, 2017; Wong Sarver et al., 2014), phobias (e.g., dogs; Farrell et al., 2021), and in preparation for dental and medical procedures (e.g., Gold & Mahrer, 2018). Virtual reality has also been tested as a strategy for providing role play opportunities (e.g., suicidal adolescent) to medical school students in their psychiatry training (e.g., Vallance et al., 2014). Although still at a relatively early stage, the rationale behind virtual reality is that clinicians can more efficiently and realistically provide a broader range of exposures in a controlled environment than would otherwise be feasible or even possible without such immersive technology.

## 1.10 Just-in-Time (Adaptive) Intervention

Just-in-time adaptive interventions are thought of as "therapist in your pocket" interventions (Balaskas et al., 2021) in that they are meant to provide psychological interventions and supports in real time and in real-world settings. These interventions are meant to capitalize on ecological momentary assessment (either self-report or passively collected through sensors) of symptoms or circumstances and push tailored intervention strategies to address issues in real time (Heron & Smyth, 2010). For example, researchers are working to develop smart-watch technology to predict aggression in youth with autism. The smart-watch technology collects physiological data, such as heart rate, and researchers used these data to determine which physiological changes are associated with imminent aggressive behavior. When the watch senses that these physiological changes are occurring the watch or other technology can prompt the child to engage in relaxation activities or other coping strategies to decrease the risk of subsequent aggressive behavior (Goodwin et al., 2019). A primary feature of just-in-time adaptive interventions is that they are meant to deliver the right type and amount of intervention based on what is happening internally for an individual or in the individual's broader environment (Nahum-Shani et al., 2015). As technology becomes more sophisticated, a goal of these interventions is to be able to predict when individuals are most likely to benefit from support and provide the needed intervention to prevent the onset or worsening of symptoms. The introduction of sensors into common technologies, such as smartphones and wearables, has allowed researchers to capitalize on passively collected data to attempt to predict psychological states based on sensor responses (e.g., movement, phone use, bedtime), in order to push interventions at the time when they might be most needed (Comer et al., 2019). These interventions are in the relatively nascent stage yet offer much promise for new intervention models and supplementing face-to-face treatment with more personalized support between sessions.

## 1.11 Artificial Intelligence and Machine Learning

Discussions about advances in the promise of just-in-time interventions for children, adolescents, and their families will likely increasingly include references to artificial intelligence and machine learning (Dwyer & Koutsouleris, 2022). Although artificial intelligence is sometimes thought of as specific to things like robotics, it actually more broadly refers to the process of training a machine or system to mimic human actions, including the potential to eventually mimic the thoughts, feelings, and behaviors that are focal to the work of mental health providers. Machine learning is one aspect of artificial intelligence that includes gathering multiple types of data from one person or multiple people generally in real time and over time. We already interface with machine learning in various ways in our daily lives, including when platforms like Amazon and Netflix start making recommendations based on our past purchases or the shows we have watched. Machine learning is also operating in the background to allow search engines like Google to guess what we are asking even when we misspell or only have a part of a word or search term. Machine learning also allows software like "Hey Siri" as an example with Apple iPhones to "listen" to and "understand" what we are saying in order to make an informed decision about what to do next (e.g., look something up, call someone, give us a reminder). As discussed in Section 1.10, these data may come from various devices and software but in the digital mental health space people are talking about including things like voice and text, data from sensors that provide information on things such as proximity to people places or things, physiological data such as steps or heart rate or respiration, and/or the types of things we are doing on our devices such as our search terms on websites. These data are then used to try to generate an algorithm or mathematical equation that tries to describe, predict, or even allow the system to respond to the behavior of the human or humans that are generating it. Of course, in all spaces machine learning requires careful consideration of issues such as consent and data privacy and security, which will remain critical as digital mental health continues to evolve.

## 1.12 Psychological Interjurisdictional Compact

**PSYPACT increases opportunities for providers to practice remotely across state lines**

In the United States, jurisdiction to practice psychology is regulated within each state or territory. In light of advances in the use of remote technologies to provide evidence-based care, many believe state-based practice jurisdiction to be an outdated regulatory model that unnecessarily limits treatment options for those in need. In response to the growing use of telehealth, the

Association of State and Provincial Psychology Boards and APA launched a taskforce to create guidelines on the use of telehealth. Part of this work included establishing an E.Passport that sets standard requirements to practice and introduced legislation that would allow states to enter a compact to allow providers in participating states to practice across state lines. This work led to the creation of the Psychological Interjurisdictional Compact (PSYPACT), an interstate compact (currently recognized across roughly half of the states in the United States) that facilitates the practice of psychology across state boundaries. Like other aspects of the digital mental health space, COVID-19 likely expedited the enactment of PSYPACT legislation in many states. If enacted in your state, PSYPACT means that psychologists licensed in that state can apply to practice remotely via technology and/or temporarily in person in other PSYPACT states. Although passed as one piece of legislation the application, procedure, and costs for each are currently distinct. To practice remotely across state lines, psychologists who are licensed in a PSYPACT-participating state are able to apply for and obtain the Association of State and Provincial Psychology Boards' E.Passport and the Authority to Practice Interjurisdictional Telepsychology from the PSYPACT Commission. To maintain the E.Passport, providers must demonstrate ongoing continuing education relevant to use of technology in the practice of psychology. To conduct temporary in-person practice, psychologists who are licensed in a PSYPACT-participating state can apply for and obtain both the Association of State and Provincial Psychology Boards' Interjurisdictional Practice Certificate and the Temporary Authorization to Practice. For more details about PSYPACT, providers can visit www.psypact.org. Examples of digital mental health tools are listed in Box 1; relevant standards and legislation are listed in Box 2.

**Box 1**
**Examples of Digital Mental Health Tools**

**Telemental health** generally refers to the use of a video and audio data to facilitate therapist-led, real-time mental health care. Most providers are likely familiar with telehealth at this point given the mass transition necessary during the COVID-19 pandemic. Although telemental health was not a dominant mode of mental health care delivery prior to COVID-19, it has now entered the clinical mainstream.

**Mental health apps** or applications are software programs designed to provide psychoeducation, monitoring, and/or skills designed to target one or more mental health concerns. This broad category of mental health apps is typically available direct to the user through various app stores and can be used on various devices including computers and mobile phones. Although thousands of mental health apps are available that claim to target a range of mental health-related issues, relatively few are evidence based.

**Digital therapeutics** are generally distinguished from the broader category of mental health apps because they require review and oversight by agencies such as the Food and Drug Administration (FDA). Given the current state of this process, use of digital therapeutics is limited to those with prescription privileges meaning the vast majority of mental health providers cannot "prescribe" them in their practices currently.

**Digital games** may be one component or feature of mental health apps or digital therapeutics or the game itself may be digital mental health tool. Although providers need to be thoughtful about the incorporation of digital games given increased awareness of the negative side effects of gaming, they offer unique opportunities to engage children in meaningful ways especially if used in moderation or with other services.

**Virtual reality** typically includes some sort of headset used in combination with an app that allows the user to be immersed in a virtual environment. The virtual environment is increasingly realistic and includes visible, auditory, and other sensory cues and details. The immersive nature of virtual reality makes it particularly promising for treating conditions in which the context of the client (user) is especially important, such as anxiety and trauma.

**Augmented reality** is sort of the opposite of virtual reality and, instead of immersing the user in a virtual world, essentially overlays sight, sound, touch, or other sensory information onto the client's real-world experience. At this point, the application of augmented reality devices (e.g., smart glasses) and software to mental health is in its relative infancy compared to virtual reality but holds promise for targeting mental health issues in which clients (users) will benefit from real-time prompts, coaching, and feedback increasing the generalizability of intervention to their daily life.

**Wearable sensors** are increasingly being integrated into common devices, such as smartphones and wearables, and can be used in combination with other digital mental health tools (e.g., apps) to passively collect a range of information (e.g., sleep time). Although still used in fairly preliminary ways in children's mental health, sensors move us further toward the opportunity to provide just-in-time interventions in the context of the client's daily life. Sensors further provide the promise of providing greater support and increasing the likelihood of generalizability of treatment and progress between sessions.

**Box 2**
**Digital Mental Health Practice, Privacy, and Data Security Standards and Legislation**

**Health Insurance Portability and Accountability Act (HIPAA)** as it pertains to telehealth (or any other digital mental health tool) generally relates to how digital data (e.g., voice, audio, video, text) are transferred and stored (e.g., encryption). HIPAA standards are generally the responsibility of both the vendor and the clinician as established by a BAA.

**Business Associate Agreement (BAA)** is typically embedded within the terms of software use and makes explicit requirements for use and accountability, including regarding HIPAA. A "good faith" grace period was extended at the start of COVID-19, but ongoing awareness and education regarding the HIPAA compliance of various apps is essential.

**Health Information Technology for Economic and Clinical Health (HITECH) Act** was enacted to promote the use of electronic health records toward more integrative health care. HITECH includes a mandate for privacy and security associated with the electronic transmission of health information, including enforcement of HIPAA rules. Although focused initially on electronic health records, companies that support videoconferencing and other digital mental health tools typically refer to both HIPAA and HITECH in their terms of use.

**Psychology Interjurisdictional Compact (PSYPACT)** is an interstate compact that aims to facilitate the practice of psychology across state boundaries. If enacted in your state, PSYPACT means that psychologists licensed in that state can apply to practice remotely via technology and/or temporarily in person in other PSYPACT states. Providers should refer to their state's licensing body regarding PSYPACT membership and requirements, which may include specific continuing education requirements in the telemental health.

# 2

# Theories and Models

Although research on the incorporation of digital tools into mental health care has proliferated, there has been relatively little attention to theory to guide this work (e.g., Glanz et al., 2008; Naslund et al., 2019; Riley et al., 2011). This remains the case in spite of data to suggest that interventions informed and guided by theory are more efficacious than those that are not (Glanz & Bishop, 2010; Naslund et al., 2017). We believe that emphasis on theory is equally relevant for children's mental health providers who incorporate digital tools into their practice. As we will discuss in more detail in the next chapter on assessment and treatment planning, case conceptualization should guide the clinical approach that clinicians take to clinical care as well as decision making regarding the use of digital tools in clinical care with children and families. To orient that discussion and contextualize those considerations, we start broadly and then try to provide more specific examples of how theory has guided the design and development of digital mental health tools, use and efficacy testing, and efforts toward dissemination and implementation.

**Theory should guide if and how technology is used in mental health**

## 2.1 Evidence-Based Practice

A chapter on theory relevant to digital mental health may benefit by starting with a broader focus on evidence-based practice. As defined by the American Psychological Association (APA, 2006), "Evidence-based practice in psychology (EBPP) is the integration of the best available research with clinical expertise in the context of patient characteristics, culture, and preferences." The APA task force report goes on to highlight two criteria for evaluating treatments: *efficacy* (i.e., scientific evaluation of whether a treatment works) and *clinical utility* (i.e., acceptability, feasibility, generalizability). The task force acknowledges that a range of methods may be used to determine efficacy, ranging from systematic clinical observation and case studies to quasi-experimental and experimental designs. Although the randomized controlled trial remains the gold standard in treatment outcome research, the APA task force emphasizes the importance of scientists and clinicians using clinical judgment to evaluate the utility of an empirically supported intervention for a particular individual, culture, or setting. In addition, mixed methods and qualitative research are playing an increasingly valued role in evaluating the acceptability and cultural fit of various evidence-based practices.

**Evidence-based practice integrates efficacy data and clinical expertise**

In the case of digital mental health, there are several ongoing conversations that relate to evidence-based practice. For example, can we assume that the evidence base for a standard in-person treatment for children's anxiety should also confer to delivery of the same treatment via telehealth? Similarly, if we develop and test a mobile app to enhance one example of a family of evidence-based treatments such as behavioral parent training for early onset behavior disorders, can we assume that a mobile app should work equally effectively with other examples? We assume that such issues will continue to be debated and explored by granting agencies and researchers alike as clinicians must move ahead making decisions about the incorporation and use of digital tools in their practice. As a final example, we noted earlier those criteria used by the FDA to evaluate digital therapeutics, in particular, may vary from the standards adopted and used by clinical scientists. As such, we highlight relevant and representative theories and models in this chapter (see Box 3), as well as the role of idiographic assessment and case conceptualization in assessment and treatment planning in the next chapter, to guide such provider decision making on a case-by-case basis.

### 2.1.1 Cognitive and Behavioral Theories

**Most digital tools are informed by cognitive behavioral theory and practice elements**

Our clinical and research training is grounded in cognitive and behavioral theories. At the broadest level this means that we believe that thoughts, feelings, and behaviors are interconnected, which has implications for the etiology, maintenance, and treatment of children's symptoms and disorders. Cognitive and behavioral theories underlie many of the field's evidence-based treatments for children and families, as reflected in the effective child therapy list maintained by the Society of Clinical Child and Adolescent Psychology (APA, Division 53). This list includes both evidence-based cognitive (e.g., identifying and challenging automatic thoughts) and behavioral (e.g., modeling and reinforcement) practice elements to evidence-based interventions grounded in behavioral (e.g., behavioral parent training), cognitive behavioral (e.g., trauma-focused cognitive-behavioral therapy [TF-CBT]), and broader (e.g., dialectical behavioral therapy, interpersonal therapy) theoretical models and approaches. Given that the evidence base for many of our interventions are grounded in cognitive, behavioral, and related theories, they are evident in existing digital tools as well (see Andersson, 2014; Fairburn & Patel, 2017 for reviews). For example, the TF-CBT treatment developers created a freely available app, TF-CBT Triangle of Life app, to aid in the cognitive processing aspects of the intervention. This is just one example of many apps that have been developed specifically to enhance existing evidence-based interventions.

That said, a specific digital tool does not necessarily need to be available for a provider to incorporate digital tools into practice. For example, a common behavioral principle is self-monitoring, such as tracking daily symptom change, sleep, or problematic behaviors or emotions. Data show that monitoring one's behavior is useful for assessment as well as treatment. In

**Box 3**
**Theories Informing Evidence-Based Digital Mental Health**

**Cognitive and behavioral theories** together describe a theoretical framework and approach to treatment that is grounded in the central premise that thoughts, feelings, and behaviors are interconnected. Cognitive and behavioral theory underlies many evidence-based treatments for children and families, which also inform digital mental health tools. Digital tools offer new opportunities for clients to use and engage with CBT techniques, including routine but important things like mood tracking and other types of self-monitoring.

**Health behavior models** are a group of models that together theorize that behavior change occurs when an individual believes that the pros outweigh the cons of change, they have the necessary support for change, and they can overcome barriers to change. Digital tools, in turn, can provide additional opportunities to provide psychoeducation regarding the advantages of a particular skill; for example, support engagement in and use of that skill, and track and problem-solving challenges to using that skill.

**Technology acceptance model** extends health behavior models by proposing that whether a client uses a digital mental health tool is determined by how much they think it will be useful and helpful. This highlights how important it is for clinicians to have solid rationales for proposing the use of a digital tool with their client and feel comfortable and confident using it themselves.

**Implementation models** generally focus how to facilitate, as well as what gets in the way of, the use of evidence-based interventions by clinicians in frontline service settings. In digital mental health, implementation efforts include considering barriers to the uptake of digital tools in various mental health care settings, strategies to support clinicians using digital tools, and the decision making regarding which clients to support, which digital tool, and when to maximize care.

**User-centered design** involves an iterative design and development process that involves all key stakeholders or end users at each stage. In the case of digital mental health for children, this may include administrators at agencies serving children, the practitioners who work there, and the child and family clients that they serve. The goal of user-centered design is to create digital tools that are desirable for the intended users, so that it can quickly and easily be adopted and integrated into mental health care and related settings serving children.

standard practice, children and families are provided worksheets or asked to create their own trackers to promote self-monitoring; however, as is common with many homework assignments, clients commonly forget to engage in any assigned homework, and self-monitoring is no exception. Digital technology can be used to help streamline self-monitoring. This can include basic technological interventions like helping clients with mobile phones use the list function and alarms or reminders to engage in self-monitoring at specific, most convenient, or useful times of day. Additionally, several mood-tracking apps have been developed to make tracking easier for children and adolescents, including Moodtrack Diary and Emotionary. These apps often allow providers to help their clients personalize the trackers to focus on emotions or behaviors most relevant to care. Finally, commonly used wearable devices, such as smart watches and Fitbit devices can be leveraged to monitor things such as sleep and exercise that are often targets of intervention.

## 2.2 Health Behavior Models

**Health behavior models suggest digital mental health tools can motivate behavior change**

Health behavior models include elements of the aforementioned theory, but also include new constructs. In a thorough review of the literature, Naslund and colleagues (2017) summarized a range of health behavior models relevant to digital mental health focusing particularly on the health belief model (Champion & Skinner, 2008), theory of planned behavior (Ajzen, 1991), transtheoretical model (Prochaska et al., 2015), and social cognitive theory (Bandura, 1998; McAlister et al., 2008). Much more detail about these and other health behavior models can be found elsewhere (e.g., Glanz et al., 2008); however, we follow Naslund and colleagues' lead by focusing on the constructs common across these theories as this approach seems most relevant to clinicians entering or working in the digital mental health space. Very broadly then, health behavior models collectively posit that behavior change occurs when an individual believes that the advantages of behavior change outweigh the disadvantages, has confidence that they have the examples, skills, and support needed to change, and the capacity to recognize and overcome barriers. Thus, if a clinician were to use health behavior models to guide their incorporation of digital mental health into social skills treatment, they would consider, for example, if and how the digital tool may provide psychoeducation regarding the advantages of social skills treatment (e.g., links between peer relationships and children's mental health), modeling of, feedback on, and support of social skills (e.g., skills video, interactive game), and prediction, tracking, and problem-solving of challenges (e.g., daily surveys, tailored feedback).

## 2.3 Technology Acceptance Model

The technology acceptance model (TAM) extends the theory of reasoned action (Ajzen & Fishbein, 1980) to posit that whether or not an individual uses technology is determined at least in part by how much they believe that the technology will be easy to use and helpful (Davis, 1989; also see King & He, 2006 for a review). The TAM has been applied across technologies, settings, and populations, including clinical populations (Rahimi et al., 2018). This model suggests that for digital tools to be successfully incorporated into practice and used by clients, clinicians should have strong rationales for incorporating these tools and feel comfortable and confident in sharing this rationale with clients. Clinicians should also be familiar with the digital tools and be able to adequately describe why they are recommending their use and offer guidance on how to use the different functionality. This should enhance the client experience with the tools and, in turn, increase the likelihood that clients engage in and with these tools. This model also suggests that both provider and client attitudes toward technology may influence the likelihood that they are used. We describe the importance of attitudes, as well as tools to assess attitudes toward technology, in Chapter 3.

## 2.4 Implementation Models

Digital mental health tools can help bridge the research-to-practice gap by making evidence-based interventions more easily accessible and by helping providers deliver high-quality care. Excitement for these tools stem from their ability to transport intervention components into the daily lives of those who need them the most. They also offer the potential to help guide clinical care and streamline the delivery of evidence-based care by providing clinicians with built-in and easy-to-access support. Although digital mental health tools were proposed to help with the implementation and dissemination of evidence-based practice, they often introduce new challenges. That is, like other advances in mental health science, research on digital mental health tools progressed with a focus on demonstrating efficacy in highly controlled research trials. There has been less attention in digital mental health research, however, to if, how, and in what ways digital mental health tools can be incorporated into, and thus effectively implemented into, mental health care settings (see Anton & Jones, 2017; Graham et al., 2020 for reviews). With this in mind, it is perhaps not surprising then that there has been relatively poor uptake and use of digital tools by mental health providers in mental health care. As a result, the field is yet again at a crossroads at which the translation of scientific advances is challenged by the same research-to-practice gap scientists and policy makers set out to address with digital mental health tools in the first place.

**Providers and organizations should consider barriers and facilitators to the adoption of digital tools**

In mental health broadly, implementation science is a broad approach that focuses on the barriers and facilitators to the adoption and sustained use of evidence-based interventions by clinicians in front-line service settings. There has been increased focus on implementation strategies to help promote the adoption and use of these tools (see Box 4). These include exploring the pros and cons of adopting a digital mental health tool (or tools) as they relate to the setting, providers, and/or clients. Then, if the decision is to adopt a digital mental health tool, you must consider for whom, when, and how the tool will be used in clinical decision making and the treatment process. Finally, providers and the administrators in the settings in which providers are working must consider both clinician- and organization-level barriers to adoption and

**Box 4**
**Implementation Considerations in Digital Mental Health**

- Consider pros and cons of digital mental health tool(s) for setting, providers, and clients.
- Consider for whom, how, and when the tool will be used in clinical decision making and treatment.
- Consider clinician- and organization-level barriers to adoption and sustained use, including access to digital mental health tools, preparation and support for data security, privacy, and use, and if and how providers can and will be reimbursed.
- Consider the cost-effectiveness of integrating digital tools, including reduction in number of sessions required for clinically significant change.

sustained use (Anton & Jones, 2017). For example, while videoconferencing may now be fairly standard in the age of COVID-19 and beyond, clinicians are less likely to have access or funding to support the use of other digital mental health tools (e.g., apps, wearables, virtual reality). Similarly, clinicians and the agencies with which they work may not be prepared to handle the IT and data security inherent in digital approaches (e.g., HIPAA, HITECH). Although reimbursement policies have changed to allow for remote services via videoconference during COVID-19, it is still unclear if providers will be reimbursed for using all digital tools or which ones in the future.

**Clinical Pearl**
Reimbursement Considerations in Digital Mental Health

Some data show that technology-enhanced treatment models can save therapist and client time by reducing the number of in-person sessions required for symptom improvement (Jones et al., 2014, 2021; Self-Brown et al., 2017). Such approaches have the potential to be cost-effective for insurance companies; however, it is less clear if and how insurance companies will respond to such data with regard to therapist tracking and billing for the time they spend engaging with the technology (e.g., reviewing client symptom tracking, survey responses, or home practice videos prior to the next session). Policies and decision-making around reimbursement for digital tools will also influence their adoption and use therapeutics. That is, the prescription of FDA cleared digital therapeutics is currently limited to providers with prescription privileges, meaning that the vast majority of mental health providers at least currently cannot incorporate them into assessment or treatment planning with their child clients or their families.

## 2.5 User-Centered Design

**Try to select tools developed in collaboration with providers and youth**

User-centered design focuses on the development of products and tools that are needed, wanted, and easy to use. The process of development involves an iterative design process that involves all key stakeholders or end users at each stage. The goal is to create a final product that is desirable for the intended users, so that it can quickly and easily be adopted and integrated into systems. User-centered design may be particularly important for the development of digital solutions for children's mental health, because youth often use technology differently and have different expectations related to the functionality of technology than adults. For example, youth are used to using social media that provide many interactive capabilities, ways to connect with individuals like them, and the ability to tailor their experience. Involving youth in the development process may increase the likelihood of adoption and use and, in turn, the effectiveness of these tools. Additionally, developers are increasingly involving clinicians in the design process. Although clinicians may not be the intended end users, clinicians play a critical role in recommending these tools. If the tools are not intuitive or do not fit in with clinicians' broader practice, they will likely fall by the wayside. As clinicians look to evaluate digital mental health tools and consider which tools to incorporate into their practice, it may be helpful to explore the development process and ensure that key stakeholders were involved. Apps that employ user-centered design are more likely to be adopted by clients.

## 2.6 Models of Incorporating Digital Mental Health Tools Into Practice

We have highlighted different products, theories, and models involved in the development, evaluation, and implementation of these tools, but it is also important to discuss models of care involving digital mental health. One such model is the US Department of Defense's *Mobile Health Practice Guide* (Armstrong et al., 2018), which includes five core competencies: (a) evidence base for mobile mental health in clinical care; (b) clinical integration

1. Evidence-Base
Providers should evaluate the evidence for existing tools and establish the appropriateness for use with children and families.
2. Clinical Integration
Providers should provide guidance to children and families on app use and ensure that they are monitoring use during treatment.
3. Privacy and Security
Providers should evaluate the privacy and security policies of any recommended apps and discuss these issues with caregivers prior to initiating use.
4. Ethical Considerations
Providers must work toward competency in digital mental health by familiarizing themselves with existing guidelines and staying up-to-date with innovations.
5. Cultural Considerations
Providers should consider how cultural factors may influence families' attitudes toward, or willingness to use, technology.

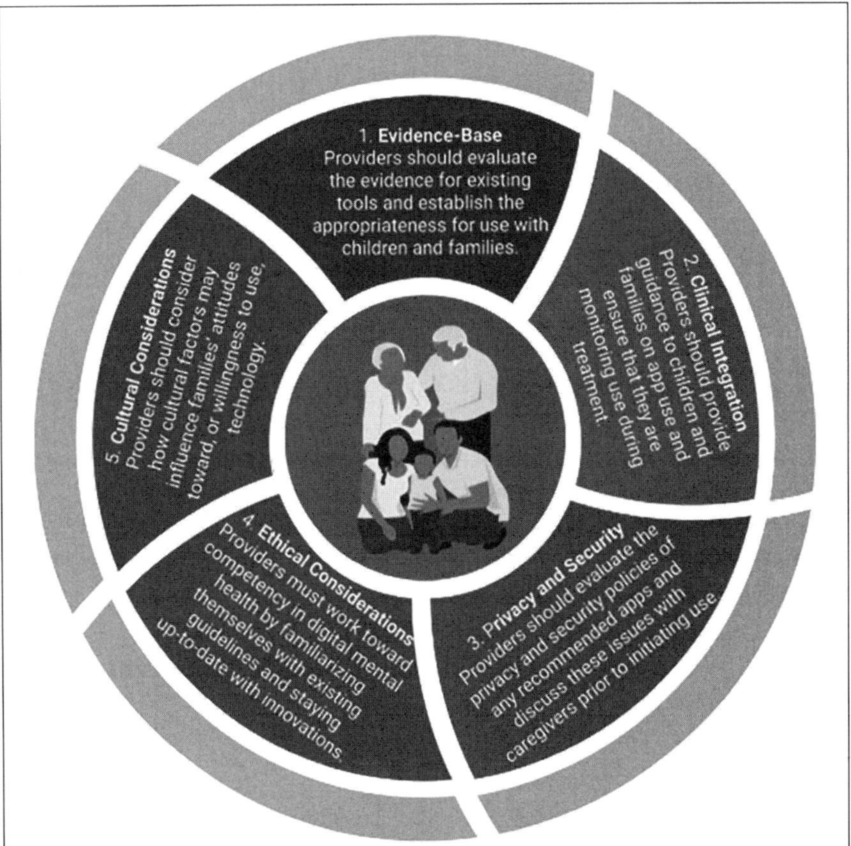

**Figure 1**
Clinical integration of digital tools into children's mental health care: Five core competencies. Based on Armstrong et al., 2018, p. 5 and Schueller et al., 2021, p. 70.

of mobile health in clinical care; (c) security and privacy with mobile health in clinical care; (d) ethical issues with mobile health in clinical care; and (e) cultural considerations with mobile health in clinical care. See Figure 1 for an overview of the model.

Although designed for military providers, this model has been applied more broadly (Schueller et al., 2021) and we believe it provides a useful and practical framework to guide the integration of digital tools in clinical practice with children and their families as well. We will use these core competences in Chapter 4 as a guiding framework and save further details for that chapter.

# 3

# Assessment and Treatment Indications

If, when, and how mental health providers use digital tools depends on access, institutional support, and reimbursement. We are not minimizing these very real-world, practical issues related to the value of clinician time, how clinicians spend that time, and what that time is worth. That said, we proceed here by assuming that a provider has access and support as this is fundamental to any subsequent guidance regarding the role of digital mental health tools in diagnostic and therapeutic decision making. With that in mind, we do not necessarily make recommendations regarding specific digital tools at least in part because the range of options will likely continue to proliferate making this book all too quickly obsolete. Moreover, we will not talk about a particular evidence-based treatment for a specific childhood disorder or pattern of presenting symptoms because digital tools may have a role in treatment plans for a range of disorders and presenting issues. Rather, we try to provide an overview of factors that may guide decision making regarding the use of digital tools, as well as the critical role of case conceptualization.

## 3.1 Case Conceptualization

Case conceptualization (also called case formulation) is not new to digital mental health, but rather seminal in the provision of high-quality, evidence-based mental health care for children and their families. Indeed, we would argue that case conceptualization is one of the most important tools that mental health providers have at their disposal. Case conceptualization is the process by which providers integrate information they have gathered on a child (e.g., diagnostic interviewing, assessment, observation) from multiple sources (e.g., child, parent, teacher) in order to create a narrative that tries to explain why this child at this time is presenting with this (or these) issue(s). The case conceptualization also provides a framework for understanding the interconnectedness of presenting issues, how those presenting issues may be exacerbated or maintained by the family, social, or broader ecological context, and, in turn, start to identify potential clues about optimal targets of intervention. We use the word *process* to describe case conceptualization intentionally as it is a framework that may and likely will change throughout the course of working with a child and family as relationships continue to be fostered, trust built, and new information and insights gathered.

**Use case conceptualization to determine if, how, and when to use digital tools**

Case conceptualization can help point to opportunities in the diagnostic and therapeutic process where digital tools may play a role in terms of increasing access to, enhancing engagement in, and/or improving (or at least maximizing) outcomes of evidence-based practice. That is, if a family has had or will continue to have difficulty accessing services either due to their own (e.g., both parents working multiple shifts making it difficult to have weekly clinic-based appointments) or provider (e.g., wait-lists, rural areas, provider shortages) challenges, then providers may start to think about how digital tools can be used to provide high-quality enhanced or stand-alone services. Presuming a family has the means and scheduling availability for weekly appointments and providers have room in their schedules, case conceptualizations may also start to reveal opportunities for technology to enhance engagement. Treatment is often hard work for families as it often includes weekly sessions, daily home-based skills practice, and commitment to continue to completion when symptoms start to improve (or are even temporarily worse!) if not "cured" entirely.

Case conceptualization may help providers determine which tools or content may help parents learn new skills at home. For example, psychoeducation via videos or online reading may be used to share in session content with caregivers who are unable to attend weekly sessions. Other digital activities may help with routine monitoring of symptoms outside of session, provide

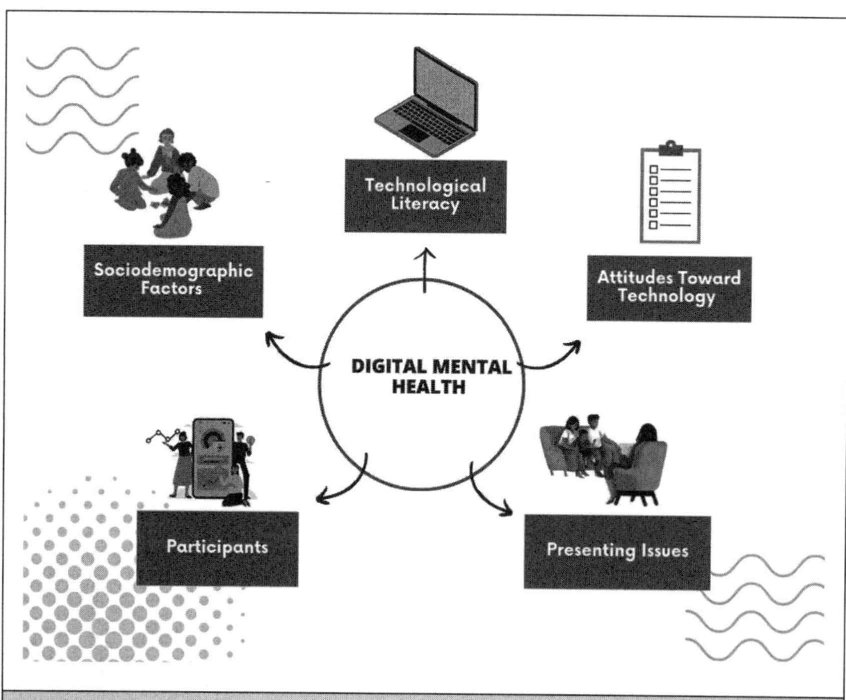


**Figure 2**
Factors that shape case conceptualization and treatment plans in digital mental health.

therapist an opportunity to provide tailored feedback on skill use outside of session, and offer reminders for homework practice or session attendance. Digital tools may also foster more efficient or robust treatment outcomes. Perhaps a child presents with a particular phobia that makes the standard of care use of exposure therapy challenging. During the COVID-19 pandemic, for example, treating a child with in vivo exposures for social phobia might not have been feasible given social distancing and associated public health guidelines. Exposures conducted via virtual technology, however, would be another treatment option guided by the case conceptualization and treatment plan. Such decisions will include considerations of the following factors (see Figure 2), which are discussed further in the next sections.

## 3.2 Participants (Parent or Child)

**Digital tools can be used carefully with parents, children, or both**

Child mental health providers are of course well aware that parents (or other guardians and caregivers) are a critical part of the treatment process. Whether they serve as the mechanism of treatment as is the case of externalizing disorders (e.g., behavioral parent training or parent management training), for example, or as coach as is more often case with internalizing disorders (e.g., anxiety), child therapy involves parents (see Forehand et al., 2013 for a review). Providers can think about who is actively participating in treatment and, in turn, generate ideas regarding whether parents, children, and/or both may benefit from digital tools.

## 3.3 Sociodemographic Factors

Access to and use of consumer-based technology continues to evolve quickly. That said, sociodemographic factors may play a role in case conceptualization and, in turn, the incorporation of digital tools into therapeutic decision making (see Box 5).

**Box 5**
**Sociodemographic Factors to Consider in Digital Mental Health Assessment and Treatment**

Age
Family structure
Geographic region
Parent gender
Race and ethnicity
Sexual/gender minority status
Socioeconomic status

### 3.3.1 Socioeconomic Status

**Families with fewer economic resources are often dependent on smartphones for online access**

Low-income families are less likely to have access to, engage in, or complete children's mental health services (Jones et al., 2016). Digital tools have thus been discussed as one strategy for increasing reach and impact of evidence-based mental health care for children and families (Jones et al., 2014). Indeed, industry data suggest that low-income individuals have similar rates of mobile phone ownership relative to their higher income counterparts. This makes sense given the digital era in which parenting increasingly occurs digitally, including the need to balance work (e.g., job searches, scheduling, communication) and childcare with other co-parents (e.g., pickup and drop-off coordination), as well as teachers and childcare providers (e.g., sick child, early dismissal). Mobile phones are thus particularly cost-effective for low-income families who are more likely than higher income families to rely on mobile phones as their primary and often only device in the home. Therefore, providers working with lower income children and families likely want to restrict consideration of digital tools to mobile apps that can be used on a particular family's mobile phone operating device. At the time we are writing this book, low-income families are more likely to own an Android phone than an Apple iPhone, given the different cost. Although some mobile mental health apps are available for both Android and Apple iOS operating systems, this is not the case for all. It is also the case, however, that low-income families are more likely to have pay-as-you-go service plans or lapses in service due to nonpayment, which must be considered in mental health service provision as well.

There is one other link between socioeconomic status and digital tools that we want to mention. Low-income children spend more time on screens on average than higher income children (Hygen et al., 2020). There are many reasons for this pattern, including the fact that low-income families may be more likely to be sedentary in general, may need to rely more on screens as a substitute for childcare, and/or higher income parents may simply limit screen time more than low-income parents. Providers thinking about digital tools in the treatment of low-income children, therefore, want to understand the role of screens in the home and the child's daily life to make decisions about the appropriateness of a plan that includes child-focused digital tools. Screen time is also relevant based on the age of the child.

### 3.3.2 Age

Mental health providers considering digital tools in their assessment or treatment planning will likely consider age for at least two reasons: comfort with, and appropriateness of, digital tools. When thinking about the latter, providers may be most likely to consider the age of the child client and the appropriateness of devices and associated screen time. The American Academy of Child and Adolescent Psychiatry (AACAP, 2020) estimated that 8- to 12-year-old children spend an average of 4 to 6 hours per day on screens with estimates at 9 hours a day for teenagers. While screens were once primarily a source of entertainment for young children (e.g., games, cartoons), the COVID-19 pandemic necessitated a shift to remote schooling and learning and parental reliance on screens for childcare while balancing work from home, home schooling, and remote mental health service delivery. As the possibility of returning to in-person service delivery seems to be on the horizon, clinicians and parenting will once again have greater flexibility and choice regarding the role of screens and screen time for individual children. AACAP recommends limiting noneducational screen time for 2- to 5-year-olds to 1 hour per weekday and 3 hours per weekend day. The recommended limits increase from there and may change over time, but the important point is that clinicians should be aware of screentime recommendations and incorporate digital tools into treatment accordingly. For example, if a child is younger *and* parents are already concerned about too much screen time, then perhaps incorporation of digital tools may focus on the parents' role in treatment (e.g., parent as coach) rather than being directly prescribed for a child.

In addition to appropriateness based on age and screen-time recommendations, age may be a proxy for comfort with technology in general and digital mental health tools in particular. Generation data suggest that millennials (born between 1981 and 1996) are familiar and comfortable with technology. Therefore, when working with millennial parents, for example, clinicians can have a reasonable likelihood of some level, if not a high level, of comfort with digital technology, which creates opportunity for the incorporation of digital mental health tools as well. Moreover, those in Generation Z (born between 1997 and 2012), which would include a range from child to young adult clients, have been called "digital natives," given that they were the first generation born into a world with instant information and connectivity via smartphones and social media. Therefore, taking other things like total screen time into account, providers can have some confidence that children, adolescents, and young adults in this age range have some familiarity with and have used various consumer-based technologies, including smartphones.

Although millennials and Generation Z will be most familiar with technology, access, use, and ownership really increased during the pandemic when parents and grandparents were reliant on technology for homeschooling, video calls with family and friends to stay in touch, and remote church services and health care appointments.

### 3.3.3 Parent Gender and Family Structure

Mothers and other female caregivers are historically most likely to seek and attend mental health services for children. This is the case in clinical trials as well, including work on digital mental health, meaning that the data to guide clinical decision making are largely based on what we know about mothers rather than fathers or male caregivers. In addition, one parent is more likely to attend sessions than both parents even in two-parent homes, given logistics of multiple jobs, schedules, and other childcare.

**Digital tools may allow other caregivers or childcare providers benefit from mental health services**

With those factors in mind, case conceptualization may lead providers to consider digital tools in different ways. If child treatment is more likely to involve one parent (e.g., a mother), then case conceptualizations may begin to guide if and how to use digital tools to include other parents (e.g., father, another mother) or caregivers (e.g., nanny, grandparent, day care provider) in the treatment process regardless of family structure (e.g., married parents, mother co-parenting with a nonresidential father, biological parent co-parenting with the child's grandparent). For example, we know that behavioral parent training is more likely to be effective if all adults in the child's life are responding to the not-okay behavior using the new skills. Such consistency is much more difficult if only one parent can attend sessions and, in turn, is responsible for explaining and demonstrating the new skills to other parents and caregivers in the child's life. In this case, a skills video series may facilitate the participating parent's ability to accurately and effectively convey the nuances of the new skills to allow multiple adults in the child's life to make changes. It can also promote consistent communication and connection outside of session, in which all caregivers can be made aware of home practice assignments and treatment progress.

In addition, there has been some discussion in the literature that fathers may be more likely to resonate with and engage in treatment if there is a technology component. That said, the relative lack of data on fathers in children's mental health treatment generally and digital mental health makes this an unanswered question.

### 3.3.4 Race/Ethnicity

Racial and ethnic minority families are less likely to have access to, or engage in, evidence-based children's mental health care. Thus, similar to income disparities, digital tools have been discussed as a vehicle to bridge this gap in services and the ways in which this will likely work best depends on providers' conceptualization of barriers to care. For example, racial and ethnic minority families are overrepresented in lower income socioeconomic strata. Thus, efforts to increase access to, or engagement in, care may rely on mobile phones to which low-income families are more likely to have access than other devices.

**Digital tools may help engage historically marginalized children**

Presuming they have access, racial and ethnic minority families may be less likely to seek or engage in services, given historical mistrust, stigma, and/or mismatch with available provider race/ethnicity. In such cases, digital tools may allow racial and ethnic minority families to seek and receive services in a less public and potentially stigmatizing way. Depending on the specifics, some digital tools may also address matching by allowing parents and/or children to create avatars, for example, that match not only their race/ethnicity (e.g., skin color and tone), but other aspects of their identity (or preferred therapist identity), including gender (e.g., male, female, nonbinary) and other physical attributes (e.g., hair and eye color).

Finally, language is another barrier to evidence-based mental health care, given that the vast majority of providers are English speaking. Digital tools that broaden access to evidence-based mental health services for children and families for whom English is not their primary language are critical to consider as well.

### 3.3.5 Sexual and Gender Minority Youth

Terms continue to evolve but we refer here to sexual and gender minority youth broadly to include lesbian, gay, bisexual, transgender, queer, and gender nonconforming (LGBTQ+). Sexual and gender minority youth are at increased risk for a range of psychosocial difficulties, including substance use, depression, and suicidality linked to bias, bullying, and victimization in their homes, schools, and communities; yet sexual and gender minority youth and their families are the focus of relatively little intervention research (see Hobaica et al., 2018 for a review). Although some providers and centers do offer specialty expertise and services for these youth and their families, digital mental health has the potential to increase the reach and impact of high-quality, evidence-based mental health care. At a minimum, for example, providers may consider the use of mobile apps that allow children or adolescents to personalize the physical characteristics of their avatar as we discussed in the case of race and ethnicity. Telemental health may further increase options for families to consult mental health experts in children's sexual and gender identities who would otherwise be difficult or even impossible to see due to geographic distance or other time or scheduling constraints. Online treatment and support programs also have the potential to increase treatment options for sexual and gender minority youth. For example, McInroy et al. (2019) studied a fairly large sample ($n$ = 4009) samples of LGBTQ+ youth (14–29 years old) and showed that they were more likely to seek information, resources, and support online than in person. Although individualized assessment and case conceptualization is critical, including understanding other factors considered here (e.g., preferences, geography), such data suggest that online assessment and treatment options hold promise for sexual and gender minority youth and their families.

### 3.3.6 Geographic Region

**Disparities in broadband access may challenge the use of some digital approaches with rural families**

Although the ubiquity of mobile phones in particular has begun to address the challenges of the digital divide, children and families who reside in rural areas continue to have less access to evidence-based mental health care. This long-standing issue is a function of a confluence of many factors including the fact that rural areas are more likely to be low income. If rural families do have knowledge of, and resources to engage in, mental health care, they often have to drive long distances to receive it. Mental health providers are much more likely to be located in more densely populated, urban, and university areas. In turn, much attention has been devoted to the promise of telemental health and remote service whether it be reaching a family in their home or via a central, community-based site where technology is available for remote-service delivery. Gains have been made with such work; however, challenges remain given that many rural areas still lack the infrastructure for high-speed Internet. Instead, many low-income and/or rural areas still rely on digital subscriber lines (DSL; i.e., dial-up) or fixed wireless, meaning that speeds rely on proximity to cellular towers or satellites reducing the speed of data transfer. Lower Internet speeds, in turn, make transmission of audio, video, and other data much more difficult. This can lead to frustrating disruptions in services or even make the provision of services impossible.

## 3.4 Technological Literacy

**Technology literacy refers to clients ability to understand and use technology tools or resources**

Technology literacy is a broad term generally used to convey the extent to which an individual is able to evaluate, manage, understand, and use technology and the digital information (e.g., text, audio, video) conveyed via that technology (digital literacy). Much like the ability to read and write (i.e., literacy), technological literacy also opens up new knowledge and opportunities for children and their families including in the area of digital mental health. That said, technological literacy occurs on a continuum such that providers may meet clients who have no or very little experience and comfort with technology to those who have far more than the provider themselves. Building upon the sections above, technological literacy may be associated with sociodemographic variables already discussed such that low-income families, those residing in rural areas, and/or older parents and caregivers may have lower levels of technological literacy, at least in part due to lower levels of access, exposure, and experience. Providers interested in using digital tools will want to do at least general screening regarding a family's access to and experience with technology at home or school or work to get a sense of the family's comfort with technology and assess how comfortable it may be to incorporate digital mental health tools into the treatment process.

For example, a measure developed by van der Vaart and Drossaert (2017) asks individuals how easy or difficult it is to use a keyboard, a mouse, and to navigate buttons or links on a website. In addition, they ask individuals how easy or difficult it is when searching for health information online to generate search terms, find sought-after information, and navigate within and between sites. Finally, they ask how easy or difficult it is for an individual to make decisions regarding whether the information they find online is useful to them and then to incorporate it into their lives. One can imagine these questions varying depending on the type of digital tools a provider is interested in using, as well as the range of digital options progressing with time. That said, having a sense of a child's or parent's technological literacy is critical before incorporating digital tools into practice and will likely also shape how and in what level of detail information regarding HIPAA, HITECH, data privacy, security expectations, and standards are explained.

**Clinical Pearl**
The Role of Technological Literacy in Digital Mental Health

If a family is highly technologically literate and familiar with and comfortable using technology for health-related information, diagnostics, and/or treatment, then perhaps only a brief overview of provider, agency, or digital mental health tool specific information is needed. However, when introducing someone with a much lower level of technological literacy to a digital mental health tool, providers will likely have to do more work upfront to ensure that children and families not only feel comfortable with use (e.g., informational handouts, guides, tutorials) but that they also understand how their use of, and interaction with, the digital tool may be linked to privacy and security.

## 3.5 Attitudes

**Client attitudes about technology shape if and how much they will use digital mental health tools**

Attitudes about technology in general and digital mental health in particular may be related to sociodemographic factors (e.g., age, income, geographic region), at least in part shaped by an individual's technological literacy and, thus, experience and comfort with digital tools. As highlighted earlier, attitudes include a child's or parent's perception regarding how easy it will be to use a digital mental health tool and how useful that tool will be. Providers considering the incorporation of digital tools into practice want to understand first, therefore, their clients' attitudes regarding technology in general as well as the digital tool they are considering. Given the active and collaborative nature of evidence-based practice and cognitive behavioral theory (CBT), we can imagine this being a conversation in which the provider introduces the idea of a digital mental health approach, the specifics of why and how they think it could be helpful clinically, and asks the client(s) how easy they think it would be to use and how useful they think such a tool would be.

In our experience at least, many families convey their attitudes clearly either nonverbally (e.g., smiling, leaning into conversation versus sitting back, arms crossed, eye roll) or verbally (e.g., "Yes! I have been writing this down on pieces of paper but having it all in one place in the app where you can see it too would be great" versus "So, you are saying you want me to do all of the other things you are asking us to do *and* remember and find time for the app too?"). Of course, even families whose attitudes suggest that they will be more likely to use the digital mental health tool may struggle to actually do so, particularly if providers are using digital tools as an out-of-session complement to, or replacement for, standard in-person treatment models – we know this about from even our most well-intentioned clients in standard evidence-based CBT for which low rates of homework compliance are a perennial issue.

To help facilitate conversations about attitudes toward technology, we refer you to the Appendix 6: Evaluating Client Attitudes About Digital Tools in Child Mental Health Care. Here we provide sample questions that you may ask a child client, as well as caregivers, about their ability and openness to the use of mobile apps in clinical care. This handout can also be adapted and used to assess comfort and attitudes toward other digital tools.

You may also find it useful to refer to Appendix 5: Strategies and Tips for Challenging and Overcoming Client Hesitation About Technology Use. In this handout, we provide a guide that you can use to organize your thinking before a session or problem-solving in sessions regarding parental or child hesitation or reluctance to using digital tools in their treatment. This handout is also designed to help you decide when to adjust your recommendation to use technology as a part of care when faced with persistent resistance from your client.

## 3.6 Disorder

Providers may consider a range of digital tools and approaches for children with different disorders and symptoms spanning internalizing (e.g., depression, anxiety) and externalizing (e.g., attention deficit hyperactivity disorder [ADHD], oppositional defiant disorder spectrum) disorders, as well as developmental disorders (e.g., autism). Again, if, when, and how to incorporate technology should be guided on the case conceptualization and based on what providers know about the presenting issue in general and the individual child or their family and broader context in particular. We provide guidance in the next chapters regarding treatment, as well as case examples that highlight approaches with various disorders of childhood. So, here we focus on two scenarios in which providers may want to weigh the pros and cons of digital mental health tools, particularly those that are child rather than parent focused.

The first is ADHD, given that there are data to suggest that ADHD is linked to overuse of technology in children, and technology may exacerbate ADHD symptomatology either directly or indirectly by serving as a substitute for developmentally appropriate learning and activities (see Weiss et al., 2011 for a review). Therefore, while providers may consider digital tools in treatment planning for children with ADHD, the benefits and potential unintended consequences of such an approach should be considered in collaboration with families.

Similarly, digital tools open a new category of treatment options for children presenting with social skills deficits, which may include children with a range of internalizing, externalizing, and developmental disorders. Virtual social skills groups, as well as a range of other digital tools, expand treatment options for children with social skills deficits by offering more convenience for parents, a broader range of peers to participate in skill modeling and role plays, and even avatars with which children can practice at any time. That said, the literature is mixed on the link between digital games and social skills, including the direction of the association (Hygen et al., 2020). For example, some data find gaming is linked to better social skills, other suggest gaming is associated with poorer social skills, and still other suggest that it is poor social skills that may lead to more gaming. There are also some data to suggest that girls' social skills may be more compromised in the context of gaming, with explanations ranging from the relationship aspects of play more important to girls may be more lacking in gaming, as well as those games are historically and culturally a more important part of play for boys than girls. As this research continues to unfold, what is likely most important for clinicians is the consideration of the child's presenting issues, gender, and broader context in order to let the case conceptualization guide the role of games or other digital tools in treatment.

# 4

# Treatment

## 4.1 Methods of Treatment

**The Department of Defense identified five core competencies related to using digital tools**

In this chapter, we use the US Department of Defense's *Mobile Health Practice Guide* (Armstrong et al., 2018) to inform our recommendations regarding the clinical integration of digital tools into children's mental health care. Although designed for military health providers, we believe the five core competencies they describe provide a useful and practical framework to guide the effective integration of digital tools in clinical practice with children and their families as well. That said, we will replace their use of "mobile health" with "digital tools" (or its variations) throughout this section to be more consistent with our broader focus in this volume. With this in mind, the five core competencies are adapted and presented next in the context of the practice of digital mental health with children and their families (see Figure 3).

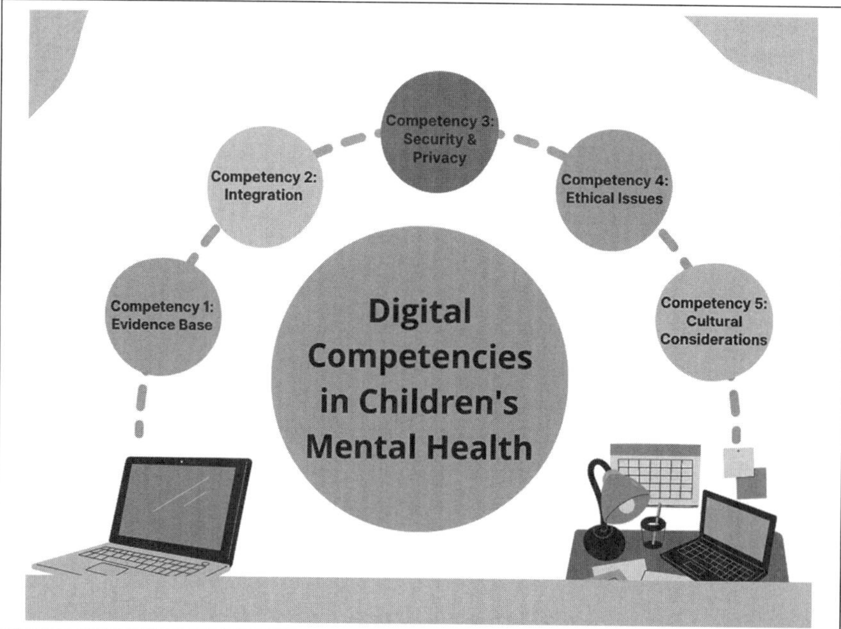


**Figure 3**
Competencies for integrating digital tools into children's mental health. Based on the *Department of Defense Mobile Health Practice Guide* (Armstrong et al., 2018).

### 4.1.1 Evidence Base for Digital Tools in Clinical Practice With Children

As with evidence-based practice more generally, the gold standard for child mental health is whether more than one randomized controlled trial has been conducted by more than one research team demonstrating that the experimental treatment yields statistically (and clinically) improved outcomes relative to the control group. While the majority of the digital tools available to providers and their clients have not been tested in randomized controlled trials, providers can approach evaluating the evidence base in different ways (Armstrong et al., 2018).

First, providers can consult empirical articles documenting the results of clinical trials on a particular digital tool or even an approach to digital mental health more generally. For example, Lindhiem and colleagues (2015) conducted a meta-analysis that included studies on children showing that those clients who received treatment via mobile technologies (i.e., personal digital assistants, text messaging, and smartphone apps) either as enhancement to, or replacement for, in-person services had better outcomes than those who had no technology component to treatment at all. Based on such work, providers may have more confidence in the potential of digital approaches to treatment.

The vast majority of available digital tools have not been rigorously evaluated in the peer-reviewed literature. We are also aware that journal and library costs may be cost-prohibitive for many agencies and providers and make keeping up with the empirical literature on digital tools difficult if not impossible. Therefore, another way to assess the evidence base of a digital tool is to search the website of the developer. As an example, Limbix is a digital therapeutics company targeting the mental health care of adolescents. Their website has a "Research" tab which describes the current stage of their research on SparkRx, a digital therapeutic for adolescent depression. At the time of this writing, they describe the results of a feasibility trial, as well as current and future research directions (e.g., a randomized controlled trial). The company also has links to their ClinicalTrials.Gov study records, which is a free database accessible to the public that includes details such as sample size, study design, and outcomes.

Given that such inquiry can be time consuming for providers, there are ongoing efforts by those in academics and industry to try to compile and evaluate digital tools. For example, OneMind PsyberGuide (see Appendix 8) uses a standardized rating system to evaluate the credibility (i.e., development process, empirical data), user experience (e.g., functionality, ease of use, engagement), and transparency (i.e., privacy and data security) of mobile mental health apps. Reviews also include a relevant professional (e.g., clinician, researcher) who is asked to download and use the app, write a narrative describing the experience, and evaluate pros and cons based on that experience. Providers can search by the presenting issue (e.g., anxiety), treatment component (e.g., psychoeducation, assessment/screening), and type of treatment (e.g., dialectical behavior therapy). At the time of this writing

PsyberGuide does not include a search criterion for age or child/adolescent versus adult. A provider could assess whether research described includes child samples and, if not, use clinical judgment to assess whether the app may be clinically relevant and potentially useful.

Even with these recommendations in mind, however, we must caution that most digital tools that providers have at their disposal will not have the type of evidence base we are used to thinking about in mental health care. Therefore, Armstrong et al. (2018) also recommend that providers consider the content contained in the digital tool. For example, perhaps a provider is considering a mobile app for an anxious child client to use outside of session to practice belly breathing. Perhaps the provider cannot find research on, or data to support, the efficacy of the specific mobile app, but the psychoeducation and modeling of the skill in the app (i.e., content) is consistent with evidence-based breathing and relaxation techniques. For example, *Sesame Street* has a "Breathe, Think, Do" mobile app that includes modeling of breathing by a monster facing a difficult situation. In such cases, clinicians can likely have more confidence in the potential usefulness of the app as a tool to remind children about the importance of breathing before acting, if this is a target in sessions, for example, as well.

It may be useful to refer to Appendix 3: Evaluate the Evidence Base of a Digital Tool for Child Mental Health. In this handout, we encourage you to consider the evidence base for a mobile app again as an example, although you could apply this checklist to any digital tool you are considering incorporating into practice. As is always important in our clinical work, we emphasize the importance of infusing your review of the evidence with sound clinical judgment regarding the quality and applicability of any digital tool for your client.

### 4.1.2 Integration of Digital Tools in Clinical Practice With Children

**Clinicians should work with their agencies to obtain support to incorporate that digital tools**

In the second competency, Armstrong and colleagues (2018) describe the five steps by which providers can integrate digital tools into clinical practice: (a) workflow; (b) introduction; (c) prescription; (d) data review; and (e) documentation. For workflow (Step 1), Armstrong and colleagues recommend thinking about the extent to which the workflow (e.g., initial assessments, appointment reminders, treatment plans) and support for that workflow (e.g., IT support) is conducive to the incorporation of digital tools with clients. For example, if an agency or provider is considering the use of digital tools broadly, or a digital tool in particular, who would be the one to do this (e.g., administration, provider), how and when would it be done (e.g., intake, as needed), and for whom (e.g., all children and families, only those who own their own devices)?

Once workflow issues are identified, understood, and resolved or finalized, Armstrong and colleagues (2018) highlight the importance of introducing the digital tool into the assessment and/or treatment plan (Step 2). For this, they recommend five steps, which we will adapt for our discussion of child mental health. Importantly, we provide only an overview here as we will use this framework in the subsequent case examples (see Chapter 5): (a) assess the child's or family's use and understanding of technology in general and the digital tool in particular; (b) describe the purpose of the digital tool (e.g., what does it target, or do?); (c) describe the key features of the digital tool (e.g., functionality, content); (d) state expectations for the digital tool (e.g., psychoeducation, assessment, skill practice); and (e) complete the informed consent and assent process (e.g., data security, provide alternatives, identify and resolve barriers).

After digital tools are introduced to the child and family, the next step in the integration of digital tools as outlined by Armstrong and colleagues (2018) is prescription (Step 3). Although the aforementioned issues (see Chapter 1) with FDA approval of digital therapeutics as "prescription only" limits provider use, here we think providers can think more broadly in terms of recommendations to the client with regard to assessment and/or the treatment. Back to our earlier points regarding assessment and case conceptualization, here providers want to think about things such as: What digital tool? For whom? How and how often? And, why? Again, we will use five key steps for integrating digital tools into practice in the case examples and thus will provide examples of prescription in that section (see Chapter 5). For now, we will highlight that Step 4 in this process is data review, which may be integrated with any digital tools with electronic health records for example in clinics when feasible or simply documentation (Step 5) in the treatment plan and homework sections of session notes.

As you begin to think about introducing digital tools into child mental health care, it may be helpful to refer to Appendix 4: Preparing to Introduce a Digital Tool Into Child Mental Health Care. This worksheet walks you through the process of introducing a digital tool into your client's care using mobile apps as an example that can be applied to other digital tools. This worksheet encourages you to consider how you intend to engage the child and caregivers in the conversation and the rationale you will provide for incorporating a digital tool, as well as the importance of addressing questions.

In addition, Appendix 5: Strategies and Tips for Talking to Your Client About Using Technology as a Part of Care provides specific prompts to facilitate a productive conversation with your client and the client's family. Finally, Appendix 7 also includes a Sample Script for Introducing a Digital Tool Into Child Mental Health Care. Of course, this is only one example, but we hope it provides a template for you to use and begin to personalize these conversations based on your own clinical style and what you have learned about your client.

### 4.1.3 Security and Privacy With Digital Tools in Clinical Practice With Children

We have talked about data security and privacy with digital tools in earlier sections of this volume (see Chapter 2). Safeguards for privacy and security will likely continue to evolve and rapidly so given the proliferation of consumer-driven technologies available to providers and their clients. Therefore, it is critical that providers are aware of federal policies on health information including the Privacy Act of 1974, the HIPAA Privacy (1996) and Security (2003) Rules, and the HITECH Act (2009), as well as any additional federal, state, and/or insurance-based policies and procedures related to use of, and reimbursement for, digital tools in clinical practice.

To provide more general guidelines, Armstrong and colleagues (2018) highlight that providers must first know whether the digital tool is being offered by a reputable source. Because there is not necessarily one consistently updated list that makes such decisions easy or straightforward, we refer you back to Section 4.1.1 Evidence Base for Digital Tools in Clinical Practice With Children. While that section does not provide definitive recommendation on which sources are trustworthy or reputable versus not, it does attempt to provide guidance regarding what sorts of information providers are looking for to make those decisions.

**Providers must help clients understand the data security and privacy policies of the digital tools**

Providers must also understand and help their clients to understand how personal information is collected by and stored on their device (e.g., smartphone) or in the software app (e.g., mobile app) running on their device. Here Armstrong and colleagues (2018) recommend providers know enough about the digital tools they are recommending to be able to explain to clients such things as permissions (e.g., is the mobile app syncing with the family's calendar or camera app?), data protection (e.g., data stored on a family's phone are not subject to HIPAA, but are if transferred to the provider), password protection and limited sharing between devices and Wi-Fi networks, setting up device location services (e.g., Android Find My Device, Apple Find My iPhone apps), and encrypting data that are being transmitting between, for example, the client (e.g., smartphone) and providers (e.g., desktop or laptop) devices. Of note, encryption relates to a range of digital tools, including email and text messages. Clinicians will want to coach their clients regarding if and how they use email or texts and, if so, how they ensure the protection of that information via encryption.

### 4.1.4 Ethical Issues With Digital Tools in Clinical Practice With Children

**Providers must consider the intersection of the APA Ethics code with a digital mental health approach**

In Competency 4, ethical issues, Armstrong and colleagues (2018) highlight the intersection of incorporating digital tools into practice and the American Psychological Association's (APA) *Ethical Principles of Psychologists and Code of Conduct* (2017). Relevant standards to consider in children's digital mental health care include: Standard 2: competence (e.g., provider knowledge of the evidence base for the use of digital tools in children's mental health care); Standard 3: human relations (e.g., including details about data security and privacy in informed consent and assent process with child and parents); and Standard 4: confidentiality (e.g., how the provider will respond to information gained through a mobile device such as a video recording that raises concern about child maltreatment). In addition, providers may consult APA's *Guidelines for the Practice of Telepsychology* (APA, 2013), as well as the increasing number of APA and other continuing education and consultation workshops and resources on the ethics of digital mental health (see the Appendix 8 for examples).

### 4.1.5 Cultural Considerations With Digital Tools in Clinical Practice With Children

Telehealth and other technology-based solutions are often talked about as tools to expand the reach of mental health services to areas and people traditionally underserved. For example, telehealth has made it possible to provide services to remote areas with severe provider shortages. However, as telehealth and digital interventions increase access to new populations, it is still critical that providers and coaches are adequately trained to recognize the specific strengths and challenges of individuals, including an awareness of intersectional identities characterized by the common context of history, culture, and community. In addition, there is an urgent need to further diversify our mental health workforce as telehealth provides new bridges to better serving diverse individuals and communities.

**Providers should consider how technology can both create and address cultural barriers**

In recognition of the importance of improving training in culturally responsive care, the final competency in Armstrong and colleagues' (2018) framework for incorporating digital tools into practice is culture (e.g., income, geographic region, technological literacy). They highlight the importance of providers' consideration of their clients' access to, comfort with, and attitudes toward digital tools, as well as providers' own thoughts and feelings about technology, those who use it, and those who do not. As there has been a shift in the field away from competence, which can suggest an endpoint at which a provider is officially "competent," we would like to recommend *cultural humility* as it instead emphasizes an ongoing process of awareness of, openness to, and curiosity about the promise of digital tools and variability within and between clients (and clients and providers) with regard to their access to, and use of, those tools. We believe such openness is critical as the diversity of our clients continues to expand as quickly as the range of digital mental tools at our disposal. In keeping with the role of cultural humility, we raise several points that may be important for providers to consider as they navigate the digital mental health space with their diverse child clients and their families, including the potential for digital tools to increase the likelihood that families seeking services see themselves reflected in the tools we have to offer.

As noted in Chapter 3, there has long been an interest in the study of matching in the mental health literature, including therapist and client matching on gender, race/ethnicity, and religion (see Ertl et al., 2019; Smith & Trimble, 2016 for reviews). Some work on matching suggests that provider and client congruence may be optimal to reduce historical mistrust, improve therapeutic alliance, and motivate engagement in, and completion of, services. To date, such data and discussions are mixed at least in part due to recognition that matching may be a consistent challenge, given provider shortages, underrepresentation of ethnic and racial minority providers, and the increasing diversity and intersectionality of our clients that in combination make matching difficult if not impossible.

That said, the rationale for matching may be more feasibly applied to digital mental health tools in which there is a growing focus on user-centered design. In the case of children's mental health, such personalization options increasingly include at least a broad representation of children and families reflecting varying gender identities, racial and ethnic backgrounds, and family structures. For example, a provider may want to screen a mobile app it is considering recommending to a family to make sure that there are characters or actors that at least resemble the child. Increasingly, children and families have the option to create their own figures or characters (i.e., avatars) in mobile apps or other digital tools, making individual choices about gender, skin tone, and hair color.

Unlike other aspects of identity, digital mental health tools for non-English speakers are still sorely lacking in part due to the cost of design and development for multiple languages. For example, OneMind PsyberGuide (see Appendix 8) has a section "Apps for Spanish Speakers" to try to increase provider and client awareness of relevant digital tools; however, none of those currently listed are for children. Such expanded language abilities are critical, however, particularly when we consider one of the original goals of digital mental health was to increase access to and engagement of children and families in services.

In addition to matching considerations, cultural humility will inform providers' privacy considerations as they relate to traditionally underserved children and families. For example, African Americans' decision to seek health care in general is impacted by the long history of discrimination and exploitation, including well-documented cases of experimentation on slaves, the Tuskegee Syphilis Study, and the first human cell line obtained from Henrietta Lacks – all without informed consent (see Wells & Gowda, 2020 for a review). This history of injustice is entrenched in the US mental health system as well (see Smith, 2020 for a review). For example, in 1851 Samuel Cartwright identified two new "psychiatric" disorders, "drapetomania" and "dysaesthesia aethiopica" that he proposed explained why enslaved individuals resisted or ran away. This long history of structural and institutional racism in the mental health care system today continues to affect children and families of color, including unequal access to, and quality of, mental health care, as well as implicit and explicit biases among providers.

Similarly, in other minoritized groups, such as the lesbian, gay, bisexual, transgender, queer, and gender nonconforming (LGBTQ+) community, there may be a similar mistrust of mental health care due to historical and systemic discrimination in the health care system. Until 1973, the American Psychiatric Association classified homosexuality as a mental health disorder in the *Diagnostic and Statistical Manual* (*DSM*). It was removed with the release of *DSM-III*; however, issues related to gender identity are still classified in the latest version, *DSM-5*. Although these classifications require dysphoria or some functional impairment related to gender identity, advocates continue to argue that these classifications pathologize normal human experiences and continue to harm the trans and gender nonconforming communities. Such factors converge to maintain and exacerbate an understandable mistrust of mental health care that may extend to digital mental health tools as well, particularly as it relates to issues of data privacy and security. Data security and privacy may also be even more relevant for undocumented children and families or even documented immigrants depending on the current political climate and fears of recrimination. Therefore, building upon our earlier discussions of technological literacy and attitudes about digital tools, providers may also want to assess cultural and historical perceptions of mental health care in general and the potential risks and benefits that minority families ascribe to digital tools before considering if, and how, to incorporate them.

## 4.2 Mechanisms of Action

Over the past decade, the National Institute of Mental Health has shifted focus to experimental therapeutics. The concept of experimental therapeutics was borrowed from more traditional medicine and drug-discovery research, and the primary goal is to identify malleable mechanisms for change or potential mediators for an intervention. So rather than just knowing that an intervention improves outcomes, the goal of most current intervention research is to understand how and why it is working. That is, what is the mechanism of action or change? Experimental therapeutics is closely linked to the idea that understanding how interventions are working will help develop more efficient, personalized, and specific interventions.

As the research evidence for the efficacy and effectiveness of digital interventions continues to grow, there is increased interest in understanding why they work similar to other mental health interventions more broadly. To date, the vast majority of research on digital interventions has focused on establishing feasibility, acceptability, and preliminary outcomes, but researchers are being challenged to identify potential mechanisms of change. This work will allow future digital intervention development to capitalize on previous knowledge of what works, why, and for whom rather than reinventing the wheel with every new intervention.

**Clinicians can use case conceptualization to guide if and how to use digital tools**

Although the research on mechanisms of change is in the relatively nascent stage for digital interventions, there are some early signs that are worth noting and that may help clinicians identify those tools with the most potential. As is common in user-centered design, there has been an increased focus on identifying and designing digital interventions to serve a specific function. Typically, in youth mental health, these functions include: (a) maintaining connection with the intervention and therapist outside of the session; (b) enhancing skill acquisition and generalization to the home setting; (c) streamlining home-based practice; and (d) improving self-monitoring. Each of these functions is thought to, in turn, improve treatment outcomes, including engagement and symptom reduction. As providers begin to explore the integration of digital tools into treatment, they should be clear on the proposed mechanism of change (e.g., why they are incorporating the tool into services and what they hope the digital intervention will accomplish). Once providers develop a treatment plan and hypotheses regarding the mechanism through which they posit the digital tool will work, they can then look at different functionalities in the available apps to select the one that is most aligned with their goals.

In addition to child- and family-related mechanisms of action, some digital interventions target provider behavior. Several tools have been developed to support provider delivery of evidence-based practice by providing decision support, remind providers of key intervention elements, and streamline the delivery of some of the more complex aspects of an intervention. These tools are sometimes designed to be used in session with the child and family and others are more preparatory and do not include features for the child or family. The goal of these digital tools is to improve providers' delivery of treatment to, in turn, enhance child and family outcomes. These tools are also often easier for providers to identify because many have been developed to augment a specific intervention (e.g., trauma-focused cognitive behavioral theory [TF-CBT]) and, therefore, are now being integrated into the broader training packages for these evidence-based practices.

## 4.3 Efficacy and Prognosis

The number of digital tools that children's mental health providers have at their disposal far exceeds the pace of research on the efficacy of those digital tools. With that caveat in mind, we attempt to organize the research that has been conducted into those that ask whether technology improves access, engagement, and/or outcomes for child clients and then close this section by considering the extent to which technology helps with the implementation of evidence-based interventions for children as well (see Box 6).

**Box 6**
**Goals of Integrating Digital Tools Into Evidence-Based Children's Mental Health**

- Increase child and family access to evidence-based mental health services.
- Increase child and family engagement in evidence-based mental health services.
- Improve outcomes of evidence-based mental health services for children and families
- Improve implementation of evidence-based mental health services for children and families.

### 4.3.1 Does Technology Increase Access to Children's Mental Health Services?

One of the best examples of research on the capacity for digital mental health to improve children's access to services is in the area of rural mental health. Rural children and families have long faced barriers to health care, including children's mental health care, due to a variety of factors such as provider shortages and associated burden of travel to traditional in-person appointments. Although there are also many challenges inherent in the promise of digital mental health for rural children and families, such as limited high-speed Internet, efforts are ongoing to increase evidence-based mental health care to rural families.

The Rural Health Information (RHI) Hub describes a hub and spoke model in which agencies are serving as spokes (i.e., they provide digital tools for children to receive mental health care) or hubs (i.e., they provide the mental health care using digital tools for students in the school system and beyond) for rural children's health care, including mental health. One of the examples listed on their website is the University of Kansas Medical Center's Telehealth Rural Outreach to Children in Kansas City Schools (ROCKS) program through which providers at the University of Kansas partner with statewide agencies, schools, and communities to both train professionals and paraprofessionals in various evidence-based treatment models as well as to provide those services to children and families directly. To date, such programs have relied primarily on video conferencing to provide remote, real-time services to children and families and, importantly, research continues to suggest that such approaches not only have the potential to increase access to evidence-based interventions but may also yield outcomes equivalent to in-person services (see Hilty et al., 2013 for a review).

Nelson and colleagues (2017) highlight that telemental health has been effectively used to address provider shortages in order to increase access to a wide age range of children and adolescents with behavioral and developmental disorders in underserved areas. Consistent with an overarching theme in this volume, they recommend that as data on the efficacy of such approaches continue to be collected, the key is for providers to use digital tools to deliver assessment and intervention approaches that already have an evidence base (i.e., only the delivery mechanism is new). In turn, increased access should also improve the efficiency of service delivery as more providers are able to serve more children and families in ways that overcome many of the most cited barriers to effective engagement in traditional service delivery models (e.g., weekly appointments, time for travel to and from appointments, unreliable transportation). This may become even more feasible with movements like the Psychological Interjurisdictional Compact (PSYPACT), which aims to coordinate cross-state practice for participating states.

### 4.3.2 Does Technology Increase Engagement in Children's Mental Health Services?

Engagement, including session attention, homework compliance, and treatment completion are perennial problems in children's mental health. A recent review of the literature examined whether digital approaches, whether stand alone or technology enhanced, increased child, adolescent, and/or parental engagement in evidence-based treatments for internalizing (e.g., anxiety, depression), externalizing (e.g., oppositional defiant disorder), or developmental disorders (e.g., autism) (Georgeson et al., 2020). Forty-two studies met the search criteria, however, definitive conclusions about whether technology is increasing engagement could not be drawn for several reasons including variation in research design (e.g., feasibility, single-arm open trial, randomized control trial) and the operationalization and measurement of engagement, including whether they were measuring engagement in the treatment process (e.g., homework compliance) or the technology itself (e.g., number of minutes using mobile app). That said, there is a line of research suggesting that a technology-enhanced treatment model can improve family engagement in behavioral parent training for early onset behavior disorders (Jones et al., 2014, 2021; Parent et al., 2022). That is, across a pilot and randomized control trial, a technology-enhanced treatment model (e.g., appointment reminders, daily surveys of home practice, skills video series) increased low-income families' homework compliance and coaching-call participation relative to standard, weekly clinic-based behavioral parent training sessions alone. The technology-enhanced model did not improve regular session attendance or completion; however, suggesting that more intensive or more personalized digital enhancements may be necessary, particularly for low-income families who are more likely to be dealing with a range of stressors that can interfere with treatment process.

We encourage you to refer Appendix 5: Strategies and Tips for Improving Client Engagement With Technology. In this section, we have focused on engagement in treatment more broadly, but the effectiveness of digital mental health also depends on children's (and/or their parents') engagement with the digital tools you are recommending. Engagement remains one of the biggest challenges in digital mental health. In this handout, we provide a checklist with prompts that aim to facilitate family engagement with digital tools, including providing a clear rationale for recommendations, approaching decision making collaboratively, attending to practical considerations such as if and how you will remind your client to use the digital tool, and addressing any privacy and security concerns, which we also address in this volume.

### 4.3.3 Does Technology Improve Outcomes of Children's Mental Health Services?

There is some discussion about asking the "right" question when it comes to the clinical efficacy of digital mental health tools. That is, in the evaluation of clinical interventions we usually ask if a new treatment approach leads to better clinical outcomes than an existing treatment or a wait-list control, for example. In clinical trials, *better* outcomes are usually defined by a statistically significant reduction in symptoms or improvement in functioning with an increased focus on clinical significance or clinically meaningful change (e.g., reduction from severe to moderate level of depression). As highlighted throughout this volume, however, digital tools are largely considered delivery vehicles for existing evidence-based interventions and/or components of those interventions. The proposed advantage of digital mental health then is to increase access to, and engagement in, treatments that we know work, but we do not necessarily need digital approaches to work better than standard, in-person, clinic-based care. Rather, we need digital approaches to work as well or perhaps it is even reasonable if outcomes are less robust but they allow us to serve more people (i.e., some effect is better than no effect at all for those children who otherwise would not have received in-person services).

With those considerations in mind, there is not yet much research resting on the efficacy of digital tools in mental health broadly and the quality of the data remains preliminary (e.g., small sample sizes, open trials with no control group, no or minimal follow-up data). That said, preliminary data suggest that digital approaches may at least work as well as standard in-person clinic-based treatments and certainly do not make child outcomes worse. Lecomte and colleagues (2020), for example, conducted a meta-analysis (i.e., quantitative analysis of pooled data) of seven previously published meta-analyses on the efficacy of mobile mental health apps, which included but was not limited to studies with child participants. They reported small to medium effects for mobile apps with relatively smaller effects for stand-alone apps relative to those with some active coaching component, with sustained effects at follow-up.

There is also mounting data that suggest telehealth interventions improve child functioning. For example, Comer and colleagues (2017) conducted a randomized controlled trial comparing home-based telehealth delivery of a behavioral parent training program – Internet-based parent–child interaction therapy (I-PCIT) – to standard clinic delivered PCIT. They found that 70% of children treated with I-PCIT responded to treatment relative to 50% in the clinic-based group, and significantly more children in the I-PCIT condition had an “excellent response” relative to the clinic-based group. Telehealth may enhance the ecological validity of care by treating children and families in their natural setting. This may be particularly as families and children are expected to adapt their routines and apply skills outside of session. Therapists can have insight into the challenges that may present in the home environment and work to address these in a way that is more difficult to facilitate in traditional face-to-face settings.

We have also shown that technology enhancements (e.g., daily surveys, reminders, skills videos) to behavioral parent training for young (3- to 8-year-old) children with early onset behavior disorders can increase the efficiency of service delivery as more rapid uptake of skills by parents results in the need for fewer sessions to see clinically significant changes in child behavior

(Anton et al., 2016; Jones et al., 2014, 2021; Parent et al., 2022). Technology enhancements also seem to help families maintain gains at follow-up, including improvements in parenting skills and reductions in child problem behavior. This is important given the well-documented regression to baseline we often see in behavioral parent training after treatment ends and parent skill use wanes over time. Finally, technology enhancements do not compromise parent satisfaction with treatment or therapeutic alliance.

### 4.3.4 Summary

Although promising, the data on the efficacy of digital approaches with children continue to unfold. However, clinicians still have to adjust their assessment and treatment strategies based on how a digital approach or tool is working in their clinical practice. Is the child or family using the digital tool? If not, what are the barriers, and can they be problem-solved or resolved? If the family is using the digital tool, is it working the way the provider expected (e.g., improving knowledge, increasing effectiveness, reducing symptoms)? If yes, providers can continue monitoring and assessing to ensure that such gains continue to be maintained or increased. If not, then providers can begin to think about why. Does the case conceptualization or treatment plan need to be adapted? Is there another digital approach or tool that may be more useful? As clinicians think about these and other questions, they may find the stepped care model a useful framework for determining if, for whom, how, and when digital tools may be most useful. In addition to child and family outcomes, however, there is additional work on the extent to which digital tools help providers themselves effectively implement evidence-based interventions.

### 4.3.5 Implementation Outcomes

In recent years there has been more attention on implementation science or how best to support providers in the delivery of the interventions that are most likely to help their clients (Curran, 2020), in order to reduce the research-to-practice gap and hopefully improve child and family outcomes. With this shift, there has been increased focus on the potential of digital tools to make the delivery of evidence-based practice easier for clinicians. Clinicians are interested in providing best practices, but often struggle to do so due to competing work demands, large and diverse caseloads, and lack of ongoing support once training has ended. The idea is that digital interventions might help provide guardrails for providers and enhance fidelity to evidence-based practice by streamlining delivery with built-in activities designed to help providers navigate clinical interactions and engage children. These digital interventions might include prompts, reminders, demonstration videos, and decision tools to help providers stay on protocol, as well as child- and family-facing activities that providers may use in session to enhance child engagement. These interventions might have particular utility for clinicians recently trained in an intervention or who, due to caseload demands, are frequently delivering different treatment protocols and therefore need to remain high fidelity to a large range of interventions at the same time.

**Digital tools hold promise for improving provider fidelity to evidence-based treatments**

Although there is considerable excitement about the potential of these tools to improve provider fidelity, the available research data are limited. SafeCare, a home visiting program shown to prevent child neglect and physical abuse, provides one example. SafeCare requires home visitors to go through an intensive training and certification process that can often be difficult for providers who are less familiar with protocolized treatment delivery. Technology enhancements have been added to make the delivery of the program easier for home visitors by adding tablet-based videos providing psychoeducation and modeling directly to parents and overall session guidance to providers (Cowart-Osborne et al., 2014). Preliminary research suggests that these technology enhancements to SafeCare reduced the time and training burden associated with implementing the intervention but did not improve provider fidelity (Self-Brown et al., 2017). Similarly, the Supporting Provider and Reaching Kids (SPARK) toolkit is a tablet-based enhancement to TF-CBT that was designed to improve provider fidelity to, and child engagement in, the intervention. SPARK was developed in conjunction with TF-CBT certified national trainers who helped identify treatment components that are difficult for clinicians to deliver and most likely to be delivered with low fidelity. SPARK was developed to improve quality of care by helping providers navigate challenging treatment components, reminding them of core principles and techniques, and providing activities and games that can be used to engage children in session. SPARK consists of nine chapters that correspond to the treatment components of TF-CBT. Each chapter has (a) a "Prepare for Session" checklist of actions for effective delivery, (b) interactive games and activities for use in session, (c) videos, and (d) provider tips to support use of SPARK. Importantly, whereas SPARK is tailored to support delivery of TF-CBT, it was built on a platform that will allow expansion to other evidence-based practices (Anton et al., 2020). Preliminary research findings suggest that the SPARK toolkit was acceptable and feasible, that providers used it at high rate, and had variable effects on provider fidelity (Davidson et al., 2019).

## 4.4 Variations of the Method and Combinations With Other Approaches

We have described multiple approaches to incorporating digital technology into treatment with a primary focus augmenting or extending more traditional face-to-face treatment. This approach certainly can improve quality of care delivery, but it does not necessarily address some of the most pressing issues in mental health care, such as workforce shortages, access gaps, and stigma. Models are emerging to help address some of these issues by using

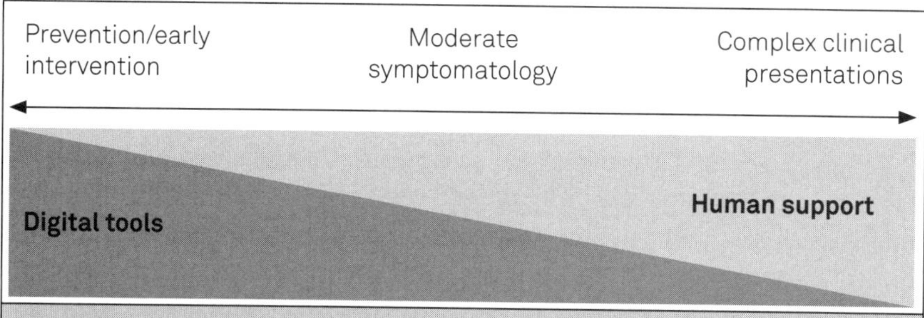


**Figure 4**
Staged care models using technology along the continuum of care. In staged care models, the level of therapist support increases as symptomatology becomes more severe and/or complex. In the early stages of care (i.e., when symptoms first emerge), or among high-risk populations, technology can be used to support population health with very little oversight by trained professionals. These models are intended to reserve the most intensive care for those who need it the most given constraints on the current mental health care system.

technology along the continuum of care from prevention to early intervention to ongoing maintenance of treatment gains (see Figure 4). These models use technology not only to augment or extend traditional services, but also add new service delivery options where more intensive or specialized services are reserved for those who need them the most.

**Digital interventions are the first line of treatment in stepped care models**

Several stepped and staged care models are emerging that incorporate digital interventions into the broader behavioral health care system. In stepped care models the primary goal is to reserve the highest levels of care and resources for those who need them the most. The goal in these models is to link clients to the most appropriate level of care that is least resource intensive first and only step them up to more intensive, specialized interventions as needed (e.g., when symptoms worsen or when the client stops responding to treatment). For example, the United Kingdom's National Health Service's Improving Access to Psychological Treatments (National Collaborating Centre for Mental Health, 2019) and Australia's Mindspot Clinics (Titov et al., 2015) have integrated computerized and digital interventions into their suite of treatment options to improve efficiencies and access to care. In both of these systems, digital interventions are considered first line interventions that can be effective for those with mild to moderate symptoms and serve as a gateway to additional or more intensive interventions, if needed.

Another emerging model that may have utility in child mental health is the clinical staging model. Clinical staging began in general medicine, and it is meant to acknowledge the progressive nature of many forms of illness, including mental illness. The goal of this system is to match clients with the lowest level of care to prevent the progression to more severe illness or even prevent onset. This is thought to be a key in youth mental health because many adult mental health problems emerge in childhood and adolescents. The goal of these models is to begin to identify youth with prodromal or subclinical symptoms and begin low-intensity interventions to prevent later symptoms and problems. These models are meant to shift clinicians' focus from treating the current symptoms to adjusting the long-term trajectory of the youth's mental health. One example of this model is Australia's "headspace," an early intervention, primary-level mental health intervention for youth and young adults ages 12–25 (Cross et al., 2014). In headspace, youth enter a screening process completed by a clinician to determine illness stage and level of care. Like the stepped care models, if it is determined that the client has low clinical complexity and low functional impairment, they will be assigned to a technology-enabled service, including Internet-based CBT (iCBT) or another digital intervention, in order to reserve limited, more intensive services for those who are most likely to need them. Headspace is a nice example then of how we can use data-driven approaches combined with personal preference to direct people to timely and appropriate services that may help mitigate workforce shortages, improve efficiency of care, and prevent ongoing mental health problems.

## 4.5 Problems in Carrying Out the Treatments

We have talked throughout this volume about the various considerations that are necessary for using digital tools in children's mental health. These include but are not limited to access, technological literacy and attitudes, and data safety and security. We will not revisit each of these in detail again but point out here that what we highlight as treatment considerations earlier in this volume do have the potential to become a problem if not assessed and incorporated into the case conceptualization and treatment planning. At the most basic level, problems will arise in the implementation of a digital approach if children and families do not have (e.g., no devices) or have inconsistent (e.g., unreliable Internet) access to digital tools.

**Clinical Pearl**
Digital Tools Are Only Useful if Children and Families Use Them

Even when individuals have access to digital tools (e.g., mobile apps), they download many and keep using very few. For example, industry data suggest 25% of apps are opened only once and most are discontinued or deleted within 30 days. If we know individuals are unlikely to stick with a consumer-based app, we also need to predict that consistently using a mental health app is unlikely as well. It is important to remember that the major goals of digital tools are to increase access to, engagement in, and outcomes of evidence-based treatments. If we cannot get children and families to engage with the mental health app (or another digital tool), then we are back where we started. Therefore, anticipating, and problem-solving, barriers to use is critical, as well as reinforcing consistent use (when possible) and checking in about inconsistent or waning use as treatment evolves.

Problems can also arise on the provider side as well. Providers have long had concerns that digital approaches may compromise the quality of the therapeutic relationship (Anton et al., 2016). Research to date suggests that such concerns are not warranted and the rapid transition to remote service delivery in response to COVID-19 may have allowed providers to see that relationships with their clients can be developed and maintained at equally high levels using digital approaches as well. Some providers will be more comfortable with digital approaches than others, however, and their own attitudes toward, and comfort with, technology may shape how they present and deliver such options to their clients. If a provider is not confident that a digital approach will be useful or whether they will be able to use the digital approach efficiently and effectively, then chances are the client will be less engaged and it will be less effective. So, providers interested in using digital tools will likely provide higher quality care if they are comfortable with the digital tools themselves, have IT support to navigate data privacy and security issues (e.g., HIPAA, HITECH), and stay abreast of evolving guidelines regarding standards of licensure, practice, and reimbursement (e.g., PSYPACT). In turn, they can likely more effectively explain the risks and benefits of a digital approach to their clients in the context of the broader treatment plan. Therapists interested in increasing their use of, and comfort with, digital tools can consider additional resources in this volume, as well as local, state, and national continuing education and professional conferences and workshops.

## 4.6 Multicultural Issues

It is our firm belief that discussions of multicultural issues should be woven throughout any volume on children's mental health, and this volume on incorporating digital tools into children's mental health care is no exception. Armstrong et al.'s (2018) model, discussed earlier, includes specific attention to cultural considerations. In addition to the examples we have provided so far that focus primarily on income and race/ethnicity, the case vignettes in the next chapter give attention to other aspects of identity as well, including LGBTQ+ status.

We have not summarized the data on if, why, or how digital approaches should (or should not) be considered or work better (or worse) with children and families based on aspects of their identity because there are actually very few current data to definitively answer such questions. Rather, we again suggest that the key to using digital mental health tools is to be guided by the case conceptualization, which includes, but is not limited to, race/ethnicity, income, geographic region, and a host of other multicultural considerations. Digital mental health, like evidence-based practice, requires the providers' awareness of the evidence base (or its equivalent), knowledge of the client's presenting issues, and the context in which those presenting issues are occurring, including culture and clinical judgment. Remember Steve Jobs's (1994) quotation we mentioned in our Preface, "Technology is nothing. What's important is that you have faith in people, that they're basically good and smart, and if you give them tools, they'll do wonderful things with them." Technology is one tool or even a range of tools that may (or may not) be a good fit for a particular provider or the child or family with whom a provider is working. Determining this fit depends on the case conceptualization and the associated range of sociodemographic, attitudinal, and clinical aspects of the case as well as ongoing continuing education and consultation for providers interested in integrating digital tools into practice.

**Digital mental health requires awareness of the context in which presenting issues occur, including culture**

# 5

# Case Vignettes

*This chapter presents examples of ways in which mental health providers can incorporate digital tools into the assessment and treatment of children. Given the mass transition to telehealth during COVID-19, we focus these case vignettes on other examples. All names and demongrapnic information have been changed to protect the privacy of the clients.*

## Case Vignette 1: Technology-Enhanced Treatment Model

Hazel is a 4-year-old White, non-Hispanic female presenting with symptoms of noncompliance (e.g., she often says "no" in response to parent requests), oppositionality (e.g., arguing, yelling, tantrums), and aggression (e.g., hitting parents and peers, breaking toys). Hazel presents for services with her married parents, Caroline and Matt, who say that this behavior spiked when she turned 3 years old and continues to worsen. Their impetus for seeking treatment now is that the day care is not allowing Hazel to return until the family seeks therapy and demonstrates improved behavior. Both parents have full-time jobs and do not have family support for childcare in this area making day care essential. They also want to address Hazel's behavior before she starts school when they fear the consequences for misbehavior will impact her relationships with teachers and classmates and affect her school performance as well.

A diagnostic interview reveals Hazel's behavior meets the criteria for a diagnosis of oppositional defiant disorder, moderate, given it occurs in at least two settings (i.e., home, day care). Her Eyberg Child Behavior Inventory (ECBI; Eyberg & Pincus, 1999) scores also exceed clinical cutoffs.

| ECBI | Score | Possible range | Clinical cutoff |
|---|---|---|---|
| Intensity | 200 | 36–252 | >131 |
| Problem | 30 | 0–36 | >15 |

Although neither parent meets criteria for depression, both parents have Beck Depression Inventory (BDI) scores in the moderate (Range 10–18) range (Caroline BDI = 17; Matt BDI = 13) (Beck et al., 1961; Beck et al., 1988). They report high levels of frustration with Hazel's behavior and admit that they are not enjoying and sometimes "do not like" their child. As a result, they are experiencing considerable guilt. They acknowledge their primary approach to parenting at this point is "walking on eggshells" to avoid her "meltdowns": They often give in to her "demands" to make life easier. Both parents report being comfortable with technology, which they use in their jobs as well as to communicate with one another (e.g., texts regarding schedules, shared grocery lists, video calls with grandparents).

Given Hazel's presenting issues, as well as the parents' comfort with technology, a technology-enhanced approach to helping the noncompliant child (HNC; McMahon & Forehand, 2003) was recommended. HNC is a mastery-based behavioral parent training program that includes weekly clinic (or telehealth) sessions that progress in two phases. Phase I focuses on skills (i.e., attends, rewards, ignoring) intended to increase the child's okay behavior. Skills (i.e., clear instructions, time-out) in Phase II focus on increasing child compliance and reducing any other lingering problem behavior. Parent–child interactions are coded in the context of child's game (i.e., child-directed play) in Phase I and parent's game (i.e., cleanup task) in Phase II to assess parent progression with, and children responsiveness to, the new skills. Mastery criteria determine progression from one skill to the next, the transition from Phase I and II, and program completion. Parents are asked to practice their new skills at home in the context of daily child's game practice, as well as to increasingly use their skills throughout the day, which is viewed as critical for skill generalization.

Session 1 included an orientation to the HNC program, as well as the proposed technology enhancements. The mobile phone app included a homework checklist for Caroline and Matt, text message reminders regarding skill practice (e.g., "Remember to practice attends today. Attends is important because it allows you to give ongoing, positive attention to your child for behavior you want to see or see more."), daily surveys of skill practice (e.g., "Did you practice child's game?"), videorecording of one child's game home practice per week, a skills video series (e.g., attends video, rewards video, ignoring video). In addition, HNC includes a brief midweek call to assess home practice, problem-solve obstacles, and provide coaching. Video calls were conducted with Caroline and Matt.

Sessions 2–5 focused on child's game as a context for practicing and mastering attends (i.e., running commentary of child's okay behavior), rewards (i.e., verbal and nonverbal praise), and planned ignoring (i.e., no look, talk, or touch in response to mild not okay behavior such as whining or tantrums). Sessions focused on brief introduction of the relevant skill, demonstration and role play between the provider and parents, and then practice of the skill with the child. Matt and Caroline decided to focus on attending to and rewarding Hazel using her "inside voice," "gentle hands" with her parents and toys, and a "calm body." Caroline acknowledged that initially attends (e.g., "You are using gentle hands with your toys") initially felt "uncomfortable" and child's game "boring." While she could bolster her enthusiasm in session it was harder at home amid the daily house, family, and work stress.

For example, one weekly home practice video revealed Caroline doing child's game while responding to text messages on her phone, paying little attention to Hazel's play, and having a fairly flat affect when she did use attends or rewards. During the midweek call, the provider was able to point out what Caroline was doing well (e.g., "You are doing child's game even though it is hard to find time!") and remind her of the purpose of child's game (i.e., boost of positive attention for child, time to practice skills). Once the parents mastered attends, the therapist noticed that Matt started saying "no" to the daily survey question "Did you practice child's game today?" Problem-solving during the next session revealed that Matt was uncomfortable with rewards (e.g., "Why should I praise her for what she should be doing in the first place?"). The therapist validated his frustration and talked about praise and rewards being motivating to all of us, including positive job evaluations and paychecks (i.e., "we all 'should' always do a good job, but are more likely to if we are incentivized"). Matt also liked the idea of "investing" his words (i.e., praise) upfront to maintain or increase okay behavior with the goal of saving his time and energy focused on Hazel's not okay behavior long term.

Once Caroline and Matt mastered attends, rewards, and ignoring, they progressed from Phase I to Phase II or compliance training for Sessions 6–8, which focused on giving Hazel clear instructions (e.g., one at a time, attending and rewarding compliance), an initial warning for noncompliance, then time-out (i.e., 3-minute removal of attention) if noncompliance persists. Here the skills video series became increasingly important to the parents as, while they had been using a version of time-out, they realized it involved lots of attention (e.g., explaining to Hazel what she did wrong, sitting on their lap, hugging her). The parents watched the videos multiple times each week to remind themselves and one another of the new time-out procedures. The midweek video call was also a useful tool for allowing the provider to help Caroline and Matt select an effective time-out chair (e.g., adult chair) and spot (e.g., corner away from foot traffic, toys, and screens but also within sight of parents).

The family required nine sessions to complete HNC, including a final wrap-up session in which the skills were reviewed and applied to new sessions that the parents could anticipate (e.g., upcoming vacation). After treatment, Hazel's ECBI scores were no longer in the clinically significant range (Intensity = 125; Problem = 10) and she was accepted back into her day care program. Caroline and Matt scheduled a meeting with the day care providers prior to readmission, demonstrated the skills that they were using and explained their rationale, then also showed the day care teacher the skills video with the hope that the skills would be used at day care as well.

## Case Vignette 2: Technology-Enabled Trauma Care

Alexis, a 14-year-old African American girl, was enrolled in trauma-focused cognitive behavioral therapy (TF-CBT), a conjoint parent–child treatment for youth (ages 3–18) with emotional and behavioral difficulties related to traumatic experiences. TF-CBT addresses core treatment components comprising the PPRACTICE acronym (**p**sychoeducation, **p**arenting, **r**elaxation, **a**ffective regulation, **c**ognitive coping, **t**rauma narration, **i**n vivo exposure; **c**onjoint sessions, **e**nhancing safety), in 12–20 sessions. TF-CBT is a well-established evidence-based practice, with extensive empirical support, and it has been shown to effectively reduce a range of emotional and behavioral difficulties, including trauma-related disorders, behavior disorders, and depression and anxiety.

When Alexis presented to treatment, she was experiencing symptoms consistent with posttraumatic stress disorder (PTSD), including insomnia, nightmares, and hyperarousal, as well as depressed mood and increased irritability secondary to sexual abuse. Alexis was referred to treatment by her case worker at the Department of Social Services following a forensic interview that indicated that she was the victim of a sexual assault. Alexis and her mother completed the Child and Adolescent Trauma Screen (CATS) youth and caregiver reports (Sachser et al., 2017). Alexis's score of 32 and her mother's score of a 25 were both indicative of probable PTSD. Alexis's mother noted increased behavior problems at home and school and noted that Alexis seemed tired. Alexis reported difficulty sleeping, including trouble falling asleep and frequent waking due to nightmares. She also reported lost interest in spending time with friends and previously enjoyed activities.

During the initial intake and first session, the therapist noticed that Alexis's symptoms of avoidance were interfering with assessment and treatment progress. Alexis was disengaged, refused to answer direct questions about her trauma, and she was reluctant to acknowledge what she had experienced. Despite the therapist's efforts to make sessions more engaging, such as bringing in YouTube videos and discussing well-known celebrities with similar trauma histories, Alexis continued to give one-word answers (e.g., yes or no). Additionally, when Alexis and her mother were oriented to the different treatment components, particularly the trauma narrative in which Alexis would need to recount details of her assault, she indicated that she was not willing to share her story. The therapist noticed Alexis often looked at her smartphone to avoid difficult conversations, and she seemed to be comfortable with technology.

At this point, the therapist assessed Alexis's comfort using a tablet-based therapy support system to support treatment that she and her mother were willing to try. The therapist oriented Alexis and her mother to the Supporting Providers and Reaching Kids (SPARK) toolkit (Ruggiero et al., 2015). SPARK is a tablet-based enhancement to TF-CBT and includes nine chapters that correspond to the treatment components of TF-CBT. Each chapter has (a) a "Prepare for Session" checklist of actions for effective delivery, (b) interactive games and activities for use in session, (c) videos, and (d) provider tips to support use of SPARK (Anton et al., 2020; Davidson et al., 2019).

In the 5 minutes prior to Session 2, the therapist opened the SPARK toolkit and reviewed the Prepare for Session drop down on the psychoeducation chapter to remind herself of the key treatment components. When Alexis and her mother arrived for the session, the therapist introduced the "What Do

You Know" game, an interactive digital flashcards game designed to facilitate psychoeducation related to trauma and PTSD. The therapist was able to select from several decks of cards to pick the information most relevant to Alexis and her family. The therapist first selected a deck of general questions that were aimed to help ease Alexis into the game and process of engaging in treatment. Alexis and her mother were able to compete by alternating turns answering simple questions (e.g., "What do you like about your family?"), and the therapist was able to keep score on the SPARK toolkit. The therapist was then able to select a deck of cards related to sexual abuse, and Alexis and her mother continued to take turns quizzing each other on questions, such as "How do children feel when they have been sexually abused?" At first, Alexis was reluctant to answer questions but as the game continued, she became more eager to answer questions and laughed as her mom struggled to answer certain questions.

In the next session, the therapist focused on relaxation skills using an interactive balloon game to facilitate the introduction and practice of paced breathing. The therapist was able to play audio that introduced the rationale for paced breathing. After the concept was introduced, the therapist and Alexis practiced by breathing along with an interactive image of a balloon inflating and deflating. Alexis was able to keep pace with the balloon and reported that the technique "felt weird," but noted that she was calmer after engaging in the activity. The therapist then went to the homework tab in the toolkit and was able to assign Alexis daily practice of deep breathing and complete a checklist of homework assignments to review prior to the next session.

During Sessions 4–5, the therapist moved into affective modulation. The goal of these sessions was to help Alexis identify her emotions, as well as different coping strategies to help manage difficult emotions. The therapist used the SPARK toolkit to facilitate a charades style game. Alexis was able to use her finger to spin a virtual wheel of emotion words. The therapist went first to help orient Alexis to the game. She spun the wheel and landed on an emotion word (e.g., happy) and then acted out this emotion while Alexis guessed. Alexis began to laugh at the therapist's exaggerated expressions and was excited when it was her turn. Alexis and the therapist took turns spinning the wheel and acting out the emotions and were able to keep score. Once Alexis got used to the game, the therapist introduced a virtual thermometer and avatar. The therapist asked Alexis to identify times when she recently experienced these emotions and rate the intensity of the emotion on the thermometer, as well as select parts of the body on the avatar where she physiologically experienced these emotions in the body. They were also able to use SPARK to create a list of coping strategies selecting both from prepopulated options as well as having the option to add additional personalized strategies.

In Sessions 6–7, the therapist introduced cognitive coping using the SPARK toolkit to introduce the cognitive triangle. First, Alexis was able to play a drag and drop game to facilitate the identification and distinction between thoughts, feelings, and actions. Next, the therapist and Alexis were able to explore the connection between thoughts, feelings, and actions. Using a series of videos that presented an ambiguous social situation, Alexis was able to select what the child might have been thinking (e.g., "I am being left out") from a drop-down list. Alexis was then directed to a follow-up video demonstrating how thoughts influence emotions and behaviors. Once that series was completed, the therapist and Alexis selected a different thought and watched the videos to see how behaviors and emotions change as a result of adjusting cognitions.

Once the therapist completed cognitive coping, Alexis constructed and processed her trauma narrative during Sessions 8–11. Although Alexis was still anxious, she was more engaged in treatment and better able to manage her emotions using new skills she had developed earlier in treatment. The therapist and Alexis had decided to write out the trauma narrative, and they were able to use the SPARK toolkit to watch a video to help normalize the anxiety about constructing the narrative and track her progress in completing the narrative. Alexis remarked that "it was nice" to see the progress she was making and made it "easier to keep going."

Alexis and her therapist spent Sessions 12–14 constructing a virtual fear hierarchy using the SPARK toolkit. The therapist relied on the provider drop downs to help guide the selection of exposure activities. Alexis, with the help of her mother, engaged in these over the next few weeks, and Alexis was able to update her hierarchy as she completed these activities. Finally, the therapist and Alexis completed an additional interactive game aimed at increasing safety.

Alexis completed TF-CBT in 15 sessions, including a final wrap-up session in which Alexis, her mother, and her therapist reviewed the skills she learned, celebrated her accomplishments and progress, and discussed strategies for maintaining treatment gains. After treatment, Alexis's CATS score was 13 and her mother's was 11. Although she occasionally still experienced hypervigilance and low mood, she reported improved sleep and was no longer engaging in avoidant behaviors. She was able to acknowledge that the abuse was wrong and that she was not responsible for what had occurred. For an additional case example with the SPARK toolkit, see Ruggiero et al. (2017).

## Case Vignette 3: Technology-Enabled Mood Monitoring

Imani, a 16 year old who identifies as female, Black, and Latina, presents with depressive symptoms (e.g., "withdrawn," "annoyed," "sleeping all the time") and associated dropping grades (e.g., from all As, to Bs and Cs), and loss of interest in activities (e.g., soccer) and friends (e.g., "lots of unreturned texts"). The depressive symptoms started after a breakup with a boyfriend, although her mothers, Nia and Hope, report that she has had some milder but similar "episodes" in the past.

An unstructured clinical interview revealed that Imani met criteria for a current major depressive episode, although she denied any current or past suicidal ideation at intake. The Revised Child Anxiety and Depression Scale (RCADS): Child and Parent Versions (Chorpita et al., 2000) were also given with T-scores of 65 on Child Version and 69 on Parent Version indicating depressive symptoms in the borderline clinical range. The family is scheduled for a month-long summer vacation in just over a month and so the provider presents a rationale for trying a brief behavioral activation approach for adolescents (Pass et al., 2018).

In Session 1, the provider shared psychoeducation about depression to help normalize Imani's experiences, including the prevalence of depression in teen girls, common factors associated with the onset of symptoms, and how these symptoms can affect daily life and functioning. The provider then began to introduce treatment and explain the different components. A rationale for activity tracking was provided, including more psychoeducation about the decreased motivation resulting from depressed mood. Finally, Imani's parents joined the session and Imani, with the help of the therapist, shared what she learned. The therapist emphasized the important role of parents in treatment and indicated that it was important that they attend sessions weekly to learn about how best to support Imani's behavior change. Imani was provided with a worksheet to track her baseline activity level daily for homework.

During Session 2, Imani indicated that she did not do her homework. Her therapist began to engage in problem-solving and told Imani that homework was key to the success of treatment. During problem-solving, Imani indicated that "no one uses worksheets anymore." Her therapist asked her to explain what she meant. Imani noted that she carries her laptop or tablet at school and often does not have a pen or pencil on her. She reported that it would be "embarrassing" to pull out a paper at school. They talked about other times and strategies for tracking including using the notes function on her smartphone to record activities at school and then logging these on the worksheet when she got home. The therapist also agreed to research other digital tools to help facilitate activity tracking prior to the next session. Next, the therapist introduced the different areas of life and values and facilitated a conversation about which of these were important to Imani. She indicated that she wanted to focus on relationships, family, and school. She reported that she felt like each of these areas had been affected by her depressive symptoms. Imani's mothers joined the session for the last 5 minutes. The therapist again emphasized the importance of homework completion and shared their plan to ensure tracking was done over the next week.

Prior to Session 3, the therapist began to research digital tools that could help facilitate activity and mood tracking over the course of treatment. The therapist began by using Google to identify potential mobile apps. She searched mood-tracking apps for depression. The therapist found an article that listed several apps for depression and reviewed each to see which had activity and mood-tracking capabilities. She found that Dailyo, MoodKit, and CBT Tools for Healthy Living, Self-Help Mood Diary all offered mood and activity tracking capabilities. None of these apps were geared toward adolescents, but the provider decided to do more research to determine if any of them might be a good fit. The therapist next went to PsyberGuide to see if any of these apps had been rated. The therapist found ratings for MoodKit and Dailyo and identified two new potential tools, IntelliCare Daily Feats and MoodNotes. Each of these apps was free to users and had similar functionality and ratings. The therapist then downloaded each of these apps to see which were the best fit for adolescents, such as including activities that were relevant to teens (e.g., completing homework, spending time with friends) and using appropriate language. She also used each app to be able to explain the functionality to Imani and her family and decided that Dailyo and IntelliCare Daily Feats would likely be the best for Imani.

**Clinical Pearl**
Picking an App for Downward Extension to a Child or Adolescent

To date, more mobile apps have been developed, tested, and demonstrated effectiveness in adult populations than those for children and families. Some of these tools, however, may be used with younger populations or parents/caregivers. In this case study, for example, the provider is using a brief behavioral activation protocol that is similar for adults and youth. The provider was unable to identify an evidence-based digital tool for adolescents, but they were able to reasonably evaluate the appropriateness of existing tools for adults for this client. When providers are making the determination of the appropriateness of a digital tool for youth it is important to consider the developmental age of the client, the similarity of app content to the content being delivered in session, the relevance of activities for youth, and how engaging the platform will be for younger populations. Many of the tools for adults lack examples or drop-down options that are relevant to youth, such as examples related to school or friendships. These tools might also seem out of touch with many of the other apps that youth are used to using. They, therefore, might not be engaging or might not resonate with children. It is important for providers to test different apps and continue to evaluate their clients' reactions and attitudes toward these tools when introduced. Additionally, many of the tools developed for adult clients have psychoeducation information or activities that may be applicable to parents or caregivers in supporting their child in therapy. These tools can be assigned to caregivers to help them practice skills that their child is being encouraged to practice, increase caregivers' awareness of symptoms or therapeutic techniques, and can also be used to help caregivers introduce session content to additional caregivers, such as other parents or teachers who are unable to attend sessions. It is necessary for providers to use these tools judiciously and consider how the use of these tools may differ for parents/caregivers trying to support their child's therapeutic process rather than clients working toward their own goals. In both cases, providers should be transparent with families about what these tools were and were not designed to do and the potential limitations and benefits of using tools designed for adults in this context.

At the beginning of the next session, the therapist met with both Imani and her parents. First the therapist reviewed how homework went over the past week. Imani indicated that she had completed her activity tracking and that being able to use her tablet and phone at school made the process easier.

The therapist then introduced the idea of downloading an app to use for homework. The therapist informed them that these apps had been reviewed for credibility and discussed the pros and cons of data safety with them. She then pulled up the app on her computer and demonstrated the different functionality of each. Imani indicated that she liked the use of emojis in Dailyo and wanted to use that app. Her parents agreed. During the session, they downloaded the app and created an account. The therapist had Imani practice tracking to see if she had any questions that needed to be answered prior to assigning the app for homework. Imani's parents left the room and using the Dailyo app, Imani and her therapist began to select activities to target under each of the previously identified life domains.

During Sessions 4–6, the therapist continued to meet with Imani to review completed activities and the impact of these changes on Imani's mood. Imani brought her smartphone to sessions, and she and the therapist reviewed her data in the app. The therapist administered the RCADS weekly to both Imani and her parents. The therapist noticed substantial improvements in their ratings with both parents and Imani endorsing scores below the clinical cutoff. Additionally, Imani noted that it was easier for her to complete activities, and that she had gotten all As on her recent exams. The therapist and Imani continued to select activities and create plans to enact and track them using the Dailyo app.

Prior to the family's trip, the therapist met with Imani and her parents to assess ongoing needs. They indicated that they felt like she had made great improvements and was feeling much better. The therapist emphasized the importance of ongoing monitoring and continued engagement in important and enjoyable activities. Imani and her parents agreed to continue to use the Dailyo app and to schedule weekly family time to review her data in the app and discuss any changes in mood. The therapist helped Imani and her mother identify changes in mood that would necessitate ongoing treatment and provided additional psychoeducation about the recurrent nature of some depression.

## Case Vignette 4: Digital Tools for Relaxation

Lucas, a 17-year-old who identified as a male and Hispanic, began seeing his school psychologist after experiencing a panic attack prior to an exam in his history class. He reported feeling increased tension that resulted in chest pain, shortness of breath, and lightheadedness. Lucas indicated that he thought he was "going to die" and had never experienced this before. Upon further assessment, Lucas reported feeling increased anxiety for about 2 months and was having difficulty managing the increased pressure of applying to college, keeping up his grades, and being an active participant in his extracurricular activities.

After the initial intake, the provider completed a semistructured interview with Lucas and his mother, Camila. Lucas and his mother indicated that he had been experiencing frequent stomachaches, difficulty sleeping, and was often worrying about his grades, friendships, and getting into his first-choice college. The provider also had Lucas, his mother, and his history teacher complete the Achenbach measures, including the youth self-report, child behavior checklist, and the teacher report form (Achenbach, 1999). Across all three reporters, Lucas had elevated scores on the Anxiety and Depression subscale and scored in the clinically elevated range on the Anxiety Problems scale on both his own and his mother's measures. Based on the results of the assessments, the provider diagnosed Lucas with generalized anxiety with panic and decided to move forward with weekly, 30-minute sessions during school focused on introducing relaxation skills and coping strategies for anxiety.

During the first session, the provider explained some of the common symptoms of anxiety and panic and provided an overview of the types of skills that can help manage stress and anxiety. The therapist briefly introduced the cognitive triangle, including the idea that thoughts impact emotions and behaviors. In the final 5 minutes of session, the provider briefly introduced diaphragmatic breathing and asked Lucas to practice a couple of times a day when he was not feeling stressed or overwhelmed.

In preparation for the next session, the provider looked up YouTube videos and digital apps to help support skill acquisition and coping. The provider decided to show Lucas a YouTube video about diaphragmatic breathing in the next session to help introduce and demonstrate the skill. They felt that watching a video may help Lucas feel more comfortable practicing in session. Additionally, the provider decided to recommend that Lucas download the free version of the Headspace app to help practice relaxation and meditation more regularly outside of session.

In the second session, the provider began the session with a quick check-in. Lucas reported that he had experienced an additional panic attack before a swim meet. The provider used this as an opportunity to discuss the importance of relaxation strategies. Lucas reported that he had "tried the breathing thing," but did not notice any significant changes in his mood or stress. The provider asked Lucas if he would like to practice again and showed him the video and they practiced together. Then, the provider introduced the concept of using the Headspace app to help learn some additional relaxation strategies and practice at home. Lucas was immediately reluctant. He indicated that he had "too much on his plate and didn't need more homework." He also expressed concern that having a new app on his phone could lead to distraction and take away time from his studying and college applications. At this point, the session was ending, and Lucas needed to return to class. The provider told Lucas that he would continue to think about it and that they would discuss use of Headspace and other alternatives during the next session.

Ahead of the next session, the provider considered the pros and cons of continuing to recommend use of the Headspace app. They also talked to Lucas's homeroom teacher to see if there was a time and private location where Lucas might be able to use the app during school hours. The provider checked in briefly with Lucas's mother to assess if she had any concerns about the amount of time he spends on his phone. Camila indicated that Lucas is very disciplined with his phone and did not report any concerns about his using an app to manage his stress and anxiety.

During their third session, the provider and Lucas spent most of the session discussing the use of an app to help support his progress in therapy and problem-solving. Lucas continued to express reluctance. The provider clearly articulated the potential benefits, including research with student populations suggesting that consistent use was associated with declines in stress and anxiety symptoms. Lucas again indicated that he felt overwhelmed by the idea of adding something else to his "long list of to dos." The provider validated and indicated that all therapy requires work outside of session to be effective and that even if it was not using Headspace there would be some expectation that Lucas practice skills outside of session. The provider also told Lucas that over time, decreasing his stress and anxiety would help him feel more able to manage his workload. The provider asked Lucas if he was willing to try it for one week and suggested that he could use time during homeroom to practice, so it did not feel like homework. Lucas hesitantly agreed to give it a try. With the few minutes remaining in session, the provider showed Lucas how to download the app and get started.

During the fourth session, Lucas indicated that he had used the app during homeroom for five minutes each day this week. He reported that he liked some of the relaxation activities but thought some of it was "stupid." The provider inquired about what he liked and pointed out similar content in the app for him to try this week and told Lucas that it was okay to repeat activities that he liked. They continued to talk about identifying triggers and other coping strategies. Toward the end of session, the provider asked Lucas if he was willing this week to use the Headspace app after school, particularly at times when he was feeling overwhelmed. Lucas continued to express concern about how this might interfere with his other responsibilities, but with some nudging agreed to use it two times after school in addition to his sessions during homeroom.

In the next session, Lucas indicated that he had used the Headspace app several times throughout the week as he was studying for an upcoming exam. He indicated that he relied on the tool to help manage his stress when he started noticing his heart racing. The provider asked if he found it to be helpful and Lucas indicated that he did. The therapist reinforced his engagement with the app, as well as his use of skills to cope with his anxiety.

Over the course of treatment, Lucas continued to use the Headspace app to reinforce the skills being learned in session and cope with his feelings of panic and anxiety. The provider continued to encourage Lucas to engage with the app by asking about what activities he had tried, what was helpful, and suggesting new activities to try. The provider also helped Lucas make connections between use of the app and his treatment gains. When challenges arose with continued engagement and use, they engaged in problem-solving and the provider consistently provided clear rationales for why continued engagement would be helpful.

By the end of treatment, Lucas had not experienced a panic attack for 5 weeks, felt more able to manage his anxiety, and had even recommended the Headspace app to a friend who was feeling stressed. The provider encouraged Lucas to continue to use the app to help maintain his treatment gains and sharpen his skills, particularly during periods of high stress.

# 6

# Further Reading

This section includes representative references to literature where child practitioners can find additional details and relevant information. The references do not necessarily focus on the treatment of children and their families, although some do. Rather, we believe each reference provides relevant information for child providers navigating the digital mental health space.

Anton, M. T., & Jones, D. J. (2017). Adoption of technology-enhanced treatments: Conceptual and practical considerations. *Clinical Psychology: Science and Practice, 24*(3), 223–240. https://doi.org/10.1111/cpsp.12197
This review integrates, reconciles, and extends the literature on dissemination and implementation, as well as technology uptake to address organizational barriers to adoption of technology enhancements. A five-stage model is proposed to address organizational readiness for, and clinician acceptance of, technology enhancements to evidence-based treatments, as well as the relevance of current adoption strategies for technology-enhanced services.

Armstrong, C. M., Edwards-Stewart, A., Ciulla, R. P., Bush, N. E., Cooper, D. C., Kinn, J. T., Pruitt, L. D., Skopp, N. A., Blasko, K. A., & Hoyt, T. V. (2018). *Department of Defense mobile health practice guide* (4th ed.). Defense Health Agency Connected Health, US Department of Defense. https://telemedicine.arizona.edu/sites/default/files/DoD%20Mobile%20Health%20Practice%20Guide-Fourth%20Edition.pdf
This guide describes five core competencies for integrating mobile technologies into health care: evidence base, clinical integration, security and privacy, ethical issues, and cultural considerations. It was developed for providers working with active military, veterans, and their families; however, we believe that the guide provides a useful template for all clinicians navigating the digital mental health space, as well as many useful examples.

Bergin, A. D., Vallejos, E. P., Davies, E. B., Daley, D., Ford, T., Harold, G., Hetrick, S., Kidner, M., Long, Y., Merry, S., Morriss, R., Sayal, K., Sonuga-Barke, E., Robinson, J., Torous, J., & Hollis, C. (2020). Preventive digital mental health interventions for children and young people: A review of the design and reporting of research. *npj Digital Medicine, 3*, Article 133. https://doi.org/10.1038/s41746-020-00339-7
This article reviews evidence-based digital mental health interventions for children and adolescents. The authors highlight that while progress has occurred, limitations remain both in terms of the number of studies, particularly with children, as well as the inclusion of children and adolescents in the design and development of digital mental health tools. Additional challenges and future directions are discussed, including the need for more attention to if, and how much, therapist support is needed in the use of the digital tools that have been tested.

Hilty, D., Chan, S., Torous, J., Luo, J., & Boland, R. (2020). A framework for competencies for the use of mobile technologies in psychiatry and medicine: Scoping review. *JMIR mHealth and uHealth, 8*(2), Article e12229. https://doi.org/10.2196/12229
A framework for mobile technology competencies was developed based on a review of the literature and the recommendations of leaders in medicine, psychiatry, education, health services, mobile technologies, and ethics. A competency framework to inform an e-culture for training related to digital mental health is proposed. Guidance regarding interactive case-, problem-, and system-based teaching to complement clinical exposure, as well as associated policy recommendations, are suggested.

Jones, D. J., Anton, M., Gonzalez, M., Honeycutt, A., Khavjou, O., Forehand, R., & Parent, J. (2015). Incorporating mobile phone technologies to expand evidence-based care. *Cognitive and Behavioral Practice, 22*(3), 281–290. https://doi.org/10.1016/j.cbpra.2014.06.002
This article delineates key considerations to guide these front-line clinicians in mobile phone-enhanced clinical practice, including an overview of industry data on update, conceptual considerations, empirical illustrations of mobile phone-enhanced assessment and treatment, and practical considerations relevant to ensuring the feasibility and sustainability of such an approach.

Ruggiero, K. J., Saunders, B. E., Davidson, T. M., Lewsky Cook, D., & Hanson, R. (2017). Leveraging technology to address the quality chasm in children's evidence-based psychotherapy. *Psychiatric Services, 68*(7), 650–652. https://doi.org/10.1176/appi.ps.201600548
This article provides an additional case example to supplement those in Chapter 5: Case Vignettes. The article focuses on using a technology-enhanced treatment model to target both provider fidelity and child engagement in trauma-focused cognitive behavioral therapy. Strengths of the approach, as well as challenges for clinicians, are discussed.

Torous, J., Stern, A. D. & Bourgeois, F. T. (2022). Regulatory considerations to keep pace with innovation in digital health products. *npj Digital Medicine, 5,* Article 121. https://doi.org/10.1038/s41746-022-00668-9
This article provides a current state of the field regarding regulatory considerations at the intersection of digital health and technology. This material may be especially useful for providers interested in more information related to digital therapeutics discussed in Chapter 1: Description, Chapter 2: Theories and Models, and Chapter 4: Treatment in this volume.

# 7

# References


Achenbach, T. M. (1999). The Child Behavior Checklist and related instruments. In M. E. Maruish (Ed.), *The use of psychological testing for treatment planning and outcomes assessment* (pp. 429–466). Lawrence Erlbaum Associates Publishers.

Ajzen, I. (1991). The theory of planned behavior. *Organizational Behavior and Human Decision Processes, 50*(2), 179–211. https://doi.org/10.1016/0749-5978(91)90020-T

Ajzen, I., & Fishbein, M. (1980). *Understanding attitudes and predicting social behavior.* Prentice Hall.

Andersson, G. (2014). *The internet and CBT: A clinical guide.* CRC Press.

American Academy of Child and Adolescent Psychiatry (AACAP). (2020). *Screen time and children.* https://www.aacap.org/AACAP/Families_and_Youth/Facts_for_Families/FFF-Guide/Children-And-Watching-TV-054.aspx#:~:text=For%20children%202%2D5%2C%20limit,about%20and%20use%20parental%20controls

American Psychological Association. (2013). *Guidelines for the practice of telepsychology.* https://www.apa.org/practice/guidelines/telepsychology

American Psychological Association. (2017). *Ethical principles of psychologists and code of conduct.* https://www.apa.org/ethics/code

American Psychological Association. (2018). *Child and adolescent mental and behavioral health resolution.* https://www.apa.org/about/policy/child-adolescent-mental-behavioral-health

American Psychological Association, Presidential Task Force on Evidence-Based Practice. (2006). Evidence-based practice in psychology. *American Psychologist, 61*(4), 271–285. https://doi.org/10.1037/0003-066X.61.4.271

American Psychological Association. (2021, August 20). *Telehealth after the pandemic: CMS outlines proposed changes.* https://www.apaservices.org/practice/reimbursement/government/telehealth-after-pandemic

American Psychiatric Association. (2021, May 27). *New nationwide poll shows an increased popularity for telehealth services.* https://www.psychiatry.org/newsroom/news-releases/New-Nationwide-Poll-Shows-an-Increased-Popularity-for-Telehealth-Services#:~:text=Nearly%20four%20in%20ten%20Americans,of%20the%20pandemic%20(82%25)

Anton, M. T., & Jones, D. J. (2017). Adoption of technology-enhanced treatments: Conceptual and practical considerations. *Clinical Psychology: A Publication of the Division of Clinical Psychology of the American Psychological Association, 24*(3), 223–240. https://doi.org/10.1111/cpsp.12197

Anton, M. T., Jones, D. J., Cuellar, J., Forehand, R., Gonzalez, M., Honeycutt, A., Khavjou, O., Newey, G., Edwards, A., Jacobs, M., & Pitmman, S. (2016). Caregiver use of the core components of technology-enhanced helping the noncompliant child: A case series analysis of low-income families. *Cognitive and Behavioral Practice, 23*(2), 194–204. https://doi.org/10.1016/j.cbpra.2015.04.005

Anton, M. T., Ridings, L. E., Hanson, R., Davidson, T., Saunders, B., Price, M., Kmett Danielson, C., Chu, B., Dismuki, C. E., Adams, Z. W., & Ruggiero, K. J. (2020). Hybrid type 1 randomized controlled trial of a tablet-based application to improve quality of care in child mental health treatment. *Contemporary Clinical Trials, 94,* 106010. https://doi.org/10.1016/j.cct.2020.106010

Armstrong, C. M., Edwards-Stewart, A., Ciulla, R. P., Bush, N. E., Cooper, D. C., Kinn, J. T., Pruitt, L. D., Skopp, N. A., Blasko, K. A., & Hoyt, T. V. (2018). *Department of Defense mobile health practice guide* (4th ed.). Defense Health Agency Connected Health, US Department of Defense. https://telemedicine.arizona.edu/sites/default/files/DoD%20Mobile%20Health%20Practice%20Guide-Fourth%20Edition.pdf

Balaskas, A., Schueller, S. M., Cox, A. L., & Doherty, G. (2021). Ecological momentary interventions for mental health: A scoping review. *PLoS ONE, 16*(3), e0248152. https://doi.org/10.1371/journal.pone.0248152

Bandura, A. (1998). Health promotion from the perspective of social cognitive theory. *Psychology and Health, 13*, 623–649. https://doi.org/10.1080/08870449808407422

Beck, A. T., Steer, R. A., & Garbin, M. G. (1988). Psychometric properties of the Beck Depression Inventory: Twenty-five years of evaluation. *Clinical Psychology Review, 8*(1), 77–100.

Beck, A. T., Ward, C. H., Mendelson, M., Mock, J., & Erbaugh, J. (1961). An inventory for measuring depression. *Archives of General Psychiatry, 4*, 561–571.

Bry, L. J., Chou, T., Miguel, E., & Comer, J. S. (2018). Consumer smartphone apps marketed for child and adolescent anxiety: A systematic review and content analysis. *Behavior Therapy, 49*, 249–261. https://doi.org/10.1016/j.beth.2017.07.008

Carl, J., Jones, D. J., Lindhiem, O., Doss, B., Weingart, K., & Comer, J. (2020). Digital therapeutics and the medical approval paradigm: Cautions for a new era in mental health care. *Clinical Psychologist, 73*(3), 22–24. https://doi.org/10.1111/bjc.12286

Carl, J., Jones, D. J., Lindhiem, O., Doss, B., Weingart, K., Timmons, A., & Comer, J. (2022). Regulating digital therapeutics for mental health: Opportunities, challenges, and the essential role of psychologists. *British Journal of Clinical Psychology, 61*(S1), 130–135. https://doi.org/10.1111/bjc.12286

Champion, V. L., & Skinner, C. S. (2008). The health belief model. In K. Glanz, B. K. Rimer, & K. Viswanath (Eds.), *Health behavior and health education: Theory, research, and practice* (4th ed., pp. 45–65). Jossey-Bass.

Chorpita, B. F., Yim, L., Moffitt, C., Umemoto, L. A., & Francis, S. E. (2000). Assessment of symptoms of DSM-IV anxiety and depression in children: A revised child anxiety and depression scale. *Behaviour Research and Therapy, 38*(8), 835–855. https://doi.org/10.1016/s0005-7967(99)00130-8

Comer, J. S. (2021). Rebooting mental health care delivery for the COVID-19 pandemic (and beyond): Guiding cautions as telehealth enters the clinical mainstream. *Cognitive and Behavioral Practice, 28*, 743–748. https://doi.org/10.1016/j.cbpra.2021.09.002

Comer, J. S., & Barlow, D. H. (2014). The occasional case against broad dissemination and implementation: Retaining a role for specialty care in the delivery of psychological treatments. *American Psychologist, 69*(1), 1–18. https://doi.org/10.1037/a0033582

Comer, J. S., Conroy, K., & Timmons, A. (2019). Ensuring wearable devices don't wear out their welcome: Cautions for the mental health care road ahead. *Clinical Psychology: Science and Practice, 26*, e12297. https://doi.org/10.1111/cpsp.12297

Comer, J. S., Furr, J. M., Miguel, E. M., Cooper-Vince, C. E., Carpenter, A. L., Elkins, R. M., Kerns, C. E., Cornacchio, D., Chou, T., Coxe, S., DeSerisy, M., Sanchez, A. L., Golik, A., Martin, J., Myers, K. M., & Chase, R. (2017). Remotely delivering real-time parent training to the home: An initial randomized trial of internet-delivered parent–child interaction therapy (I-PCIT). *Journal of Consulting and Clinical Psychology, 85*(9), 909–917. https://doi.org/10.1037/ccp0000230

Cowart-Osborne, M., Jackson, M., Chege, E., Baker, E., Whitaker, D., & Self-Brown, S. (2014). Technology-based innovations in child maltreatment prevention programs: Examples from SafeCare®. *Social Sciences (Basel, Switzerland), 3*(3), 427–440. https://doi.org/10.3390/socsci3030427

Cross, S. P., Hermens, D. F., Scott, E. M., Ottavio, A., McGorry, P. D., & Hickie, I. B. (2014). A clinical staging model for early intervention youth mental health services. *Psychiatric Services, 65*(7), 939–943. https://doi.org/10.1176/appi.ps.201300221

Curran, G. M. (2020). Implementation science made too simple: A teaching tool. *Implementation Science Communications, 1*(27). https://doi.org/10.1186/s43058-020-00001-z

Davidson, T. M., Bunnell, B. E., Saunders, B. E., Hanson, R. F., Danielson, C. K., Cook, D., Chu, B. C., Dorsey, S., Adams, Z. W., Andrews, A. R., Walker, J. H., Soltis, K. E., Cohen, J. A., Deblinger, E., & Ruggiero, K. J. (2019). Pilot evaluation of a tablet-based application to improve quality of care in child mental health treatment. *Behavior Therapy, 50*(2), 367–379. https://doi.org/10.1016/j.beth.2018.07.005

Davis, F. D. (1989). Perceived usefulness, perceived ease of use, and user acceptance of information technology. *MIS Quarterly, 13*(3), 319–340. https://doi.org/10.2307/249008

Digital Therapeutics Alliance. (2020). *What is a digital therapeutic?* https://dtxalliance.org/understanding-dtx/what-is-a-dtx/

Doss, B. D., Weingardt, K. R., Lindhiem, O. J., Timmons, A. C., Jones, D. J., Comer, J. S., & Carl, J. (2021). Issues in regulating DTx. *Psychiatric Times, 38*(Supplement), 6–7.

Dwyer, D., & Koutsouleris, N. (2022). Annual research review: Translational machine learning for child and adolescent psychiatry. *Journal of Child Psychology and Psychiatry, 63*(4), 421–443. https://doi.org/10.1111/jcpp.13545

Ertl, M., Mann-Saumier, M., Martin, R., Graves, D., & Altarriba, J. (2019). The impossibility of client–therapist "match": Implications and future directions for multicultural competency. *Journal of Mental Health Counseling, 41*(4), 312–326. https://doi.org/10.17744/mehc.41.4.03

Executive Board, 142. (2017). *mHealth: Use of appropriate digital technologies for public health: Report by the director-general.* World Health Organization. https://apps.who.int/iris/handle/10665/274134

Eyberg, S. M., & Pincus, D. (1999). *Eyberg Child Behavior Inventory and Sutter-Eyberg Student Behavior Inventory-Revised: Professional manual.* Psychological Assessment Resources.

Fairburn, C. G., & Patel, V. (2017). The impact of digital technology on psychological treatments and their dissemination. *Behaviour Research and Therapy, 88*, 19–25. https://doi.org/10.1016/j.brat.2016.08.012

Farrell, L. J., Miyamoto, T., Donovan, C. L., Waters, A. M., Krisch, K. A., & Ollendick, T. H. (2021). Virtual reality one-session treatment of child-specific phobia of dogs: A controlled multiple baseline case series. *Behavior Therapy, 52*(2), 478–491. https://doi.org/10.1016/j.beth.2020.06.003

Fehr, K. K., Leraas, B. C., & Littles, M. M. D. (2020). Behavioral health needs, barriers, and parent preferences in rural pediatric primary care. *Journal of Pediatric Psychology, 45*(8), 910–920. https://doi.org/10.1093/jpepsy/jsaa057

Ferrari, M., McIlwaine, S. V., Reynolds, J. A., Archie, S., Boydell, K., Lal, S., Shah, J. L., Henderson, J., Alvarez-Jimenez, M., Andersson, N., Boruff, J., Nielsen, R., & Iyer, S. N. (2020). Digital game interventions for youth mental health services (gaming my way to recovery): Protocol for a scoping review. *JMIR Research Protocols, 9*(6), e13834. https://doi.org/10.2196/13834

Forehand, R., Jones, D. J., & Parent, J. (2013). Behavioral parenting interventions for child disruptive behaviors and anxiety: What's different and what's the same. *Clinical Psychology Review, 33*(1), 133-145. https://doi.org/10.1016/j.cpr.2012.10.010

Georgeson, A. R., Highlander, A., Loiselle, R., Zachary, C., & Jones, D. J. (2020). Engagement in technology-enhanced interventions for children and adolescents: Current status and recommendations for moving forward. *Clinical Psychology Review, 78*, 101858. https://doi.org/10.1016/j.cpr.2020.101858

Glanz, K., & Bishop, D. B. (2010). The role of behavioral science theory in development and implementation of public health interventions. *Annual Review of Public Health, 31*, 399–418. https://doi.org/10.1146/annurev.publhealth.012809.103604

Glanz, K., Rimer, B. K., & Viswanath, K. (Eds.). (2008). *Health behavior and health education: Theory, research, and practice* (4th ed.). Jossey-Bass.

Goodell, J. (2011, January 17). Steve Jobs in 1994: The Rolling Stone interview. *Rolling Stone*. https://www.rollingstone.com/culture/culture-news/steve-jobs-in-1994-the-rolling-stone-interview-231132/

Gold, J. I., & Mahrer, N. E. (2018). Is virtual reality ready for prime time in the medical space? A randomized control trial of pediatric virtual reality for acute procedural pain management. *Journal of Pediatric Psychology, 43*(3), 266–275. https://doi.org/10.1093/jpepsy/jsx129

Goodwin, M. S., Mazefsky, C. A., Ioannidis, S., Erdogmus, D., & Siegel, M. (2019). Predicting aggression to others in youth with autism using a wearable biosensor. *Autism Research, 12*(8), 1286–1296. https://doi.org/10.1002/aur.2151

Graham, A. K., Lattie, E. G., Powell, B. J., Lyon, A. R., Smith, J. D., Schueller, S. M., Stadnick, N. A., Brown, C. H., & Mohr, D. C. (2020). Implementation strategies for digital mental health interventions in health care settings. *American Psychologist, 75*(8), 1080–1092. https://doi.org/10.1037/amp0000686

Halldorsson, B., Hill, C., Waite, P., Partridge, K., Freeman, D., & Creswell, C. (2021). Annual research review. Immersive virtual reality and digital applied gaming interventions for the treatment of mental health problems in children and young people: The need for rigorous treatment development and clinical evaluation. *Journal of Child Psychology and Psychiatry, and Allied Disciplines, 62*(5), 584–605. https://doi.org/10.1111/jcpp.13400

Heron, K. E., & Smyth, J. M. (2010). Ecological momentary interventions: Incorporating mobile technology into psychosocial and health behaviour treatments. *British Journal of Health Psychology, 15*(1), 1–39. https://doi.org/10.1348/135910709X466063

Hilty, D. M., Ferrer, D. C., Parish, M. B., Johnston, B., Callahan, E. J., & Yellowlees, P. M. (2013). The effectiveness of telemental health: A 2013 review. *Telemedicine Journal and e-Health, 19*(6), 444–454. https://doi.org/10.1089/tmj.2013.0075

Hobaica, S., Alman, A., Jackowich, S., & Kwon, P. (2018). Empirically based psychological interventions with sexual minority youth: A systematic review. *Psychology of Sexual Orientation and Gender Diversity, 5*(3), 313–323. https://doi.org/10.1037/sgd0000275

Hygen, B. W., Belsky, J., Stenseng, F., Skalicka, V., Kvande, M. N., Zahl-Thanem, T., & Wichstrøm, L. (2020). Time spent gaming and social competence in children: Reciprocal effects across childhood. *Child Development, 91*, 861–875. https://doi.org/10.1111/cdev.13243

IMDRF Software as a Medical Device (SaMD) Working Group. (2014). *"Software as a medical device": Possible framework for risk categorization and corresponding considerations*. https://www.imdrf.org/sites/default/files/docs/imdrf/final/technical/imdrf-tech-140918-samd-framework-risk-categorization-141013.pdf

Jones, D. J., Anton, M., Zachary, C., Pittman, S., Turner, P., Forehand, R., & Khavjou, O. (2016). A review of the key considerations in mental health services research: A focus on low-income children and families. *Couple & Family Psychology, 5*(4), 240–257. https://doi.org/10.1037/cfp0000069

Jones, D. J., Forehand, R., Cuellar, J., Parent, J., Honeycutt, A., Khavjou, O., Gonzalez, M., Anton, M., & Newey, G. A. (2014). Technology-enhanced program for child disruptive behavior disorders: Development and pilot randomized control trial. *Journal of Clinical Child and Adolescent Psychology*, 43(1), 88–101. https://doi.org/10.1080/15374416.2013.822308

Jones, D. J., Loiselle, R., Zachary, C., Georgeson, A. R., Highlander, A., Turner, P., Youngstrom, J. K., Khavjou, O., Anton, M. T., Gonzalez, M., Bresland, N. L., & Forehand, R. (2021). Optimizing engagement in behavioral parent training: Progress toward a technology-enhanced treatment model. *Behavior Therapy*, 52(2), 508–521. https://doi.org/10.1016/j.beth.2020.07.001

Kazdin, A. E., & Blase, S. L. (2011). Rebooting psychotherapy research and practice to reduce the burden of mental illness. *Perspectives on Psychological Science, 6*(1), 21–37. https://doi.org/10.1177/1745691610393527

King, W. R., & He, J. (2006). A meta-analysis of the technology acceptance model. *Information & Management, 43*(6), 740–755. https://doi.org/10.1016/j.im.2006.05.003

Larsen, M. E., Huckvale, K., Nicholas, J., Torous, J., Birrell, L., Li, E., & Reda, B. (2019). Using science to sell apps: Evaluation of mental health app store quality claims. *npj Digital Medicine, 2*(18). https://doi.org/10.1038/s41746-019-0093-1

Le, T.-A. P., & Beidel, D. C. (2017). Psychometric properties of a social skills assessment using a virtual environment. *Journal of Psychopathology and Behavioral Assessment, 39*, 230–240. https://doi.org/10.1007/s10862-017-9589-7

Lecomte, T., Potvin, S., Corbiere, M., Guay, S., Samson, C., Cloutier, B., Fancoueur, A., Pennou, A., & Khazall, Y. (2020). Mobile apps for mental health issues: Meta-review of meta-analyses. *JMIR mHealth and uHealth, 8*(5), e17558. https://doi.org/10.2196/17458

Lindhiem, O., Bennett, C. B., Rosen, D., & Silk, J. (2015). Mobile technology boosts the effectiveness of psychotherapy and behavioral interventions: A meta-analysis. *Behavior Modification, 39*(6), 785–804. https://doi.org/10.1177/0145445515595198

Liu, R., Salisbury, J. P., Vahabzadeh, A., & Sahin, N. T. (2017). Feasibility of an autism-focused augmented reality smartglasses system for social communication and behavioral coaching. *Frontiers in Pediatrics, 5*, Article 145. https://doi.org/10.3389/fped.2017.00145

Maskey, M., Rodgers, J., Grahame, V., Glod, M., Honey, E., Kinnear, J., Labus, M., Milne, J., Minos, D., McConachie, H., & Parr, J. R. (2019). A randomised controlled feasibility trial of immersive virtual reality treatment with cognitive behaviour therapy for specific phobias in young people with autism spectrum disorder. *Journal of Autism and Developmental Disorders, 49*(5), 1912–1927. https://doi.org/10.1007/s10803-018-3861-x

McAlister, A. L., Perry, C. L., & Parcel, G. S. (2008). How individuals, environments, and health behaviors interact: Social cognitive theory. In K. Glanz, B. K. Rimer, & K. Viswanath (Eds.), *Health behavior and health education: Theory, research, and practice* (4th ed., pp. 169–188). Jossey-Bass.

McInroy, L. B., McCloskey, R. J., Craig, S. L., & Eaton, A. D. (2019). LGBTQ+ youths' community engagement and resource seeking online versus offline. *Journal of Technology in Human Services, 37*(4), 315–333. https://doi.org/10.1080/15228835.2019.1617823

McMahon, R. J., & Forehand, R. L. (2003). *Helping the noncompliant child: Family-based treatment for oppositional behavior* (2nd ed.). Guilford Press.

Mohr, D. C., Cuijpers, P., & Lehman, K. (2011). Supportive accountability: A model for providing human support to enhance adherence to eHealth interventions. *Journal of Medical Internet Research, 13*(1), e30. https://doi.org/10.2196/jmir.1602

Nahum-Shani, I., Hekler, E. B., & Spruijt-Metz, D. (2015). Building health behavior models to guide the development of just-in-time adaptive interventions: A pragmatic framework. *Health Psychology: Official Journal of the Division of Health Psychology, American Psychological Association, 34*(Suppl.), 1209–1219. https://doi.org/10.1037/hea0000306

Naslund, J. A., Aschbrenner, K. A., Kim, S. J., McHugo, G. J., Unützer, J., Bartels, S. J., & Marsch, L. A. (2017). Health behavior models for informing digital technology interventions for individuals with mental illness. *Psychiatric Rehabilitation Journal, 40*(3), 325–335. https://doi.org/10.1037/prj0000246

Naslund, J. A., Aschbrenner, K. A., McHugo, G. J., Unützer, J., Marsch, L. A., & Bartels, S. J. (2019). Exploring opportunities to support mental health care using social media: A survey of social media users with mental illness. *Early Intervention in Psychiatry, 13*(3), 405–413. https://doi.org/10.1111/eip.12496

National Collaborating Centre for Mental Health. (2019). *The improving access to psychological therapies manual.* https://www.england.nhs.uk/wp-content/uploads/2018/06/the-iapt-manual-v5.pdf

Nelson, E. L., Cain, S., & Sharp, S. (2017). Considerations for conducting telemental health with children and adolescents. *Child and Adolescent Psychiatric Clinics, 26*(1), 77–91. https://doi.org/10.1016/j.chc.2016.07.008

Parent, J., Anton, M. T., Loiselle, R., Highlander, A., Breslend, N., Forehand, R., Hare, M., Youngstrom, J. K., & Jones, D. J. (2022). A randomized controlled trial of technology-enhanced behavioral parent training: Sustained parent skill use and child outcomes at follow-up. *Journal of Child Psychology and Psychiatry, and Allied Disciplines, 63*(9), 992–1001. https://doi.org/10.1111/jcpp.13554

Pass, L., Lejuez, C. W., & Reynolds, S. (2018). Brief behavioural activation (Brief BA) for adolescent depression: A pilot study. *Behavioural and Cognitive Psychotherapy, 46*(2), 182–194. https://doi.org/10.1017/S1352465817000443

Pew Research Center. (2019). *Mobile fact sheet*. https://www.pewresearch.org/internet/fact-sheet/mobile/

Pramana, G., Parmanto, B., Kendall, P. C., & Silk, J. S. (2014). The SmartCAT: An m-health platform for ecological momentary intervention in child anxiety treatment. *Telemedicine Journal and E-health, 20*(5), 419–427. https://doi.org/10.1089/tmj.2013.0214

Pramana, G., Parmanto, B., Lomas, J., Lindhiem, O., Kendall, P. C., & Silk, J. (2018). Using mobile health gamification to facilitate cognitive behavioral therapy skills practice in child anxiety treatment: Open clinical trial. *JMIR Serious Games, 6*(2), e9. https://doi.org/10.2196/games.8902

Prochaska, J. O., Redding, C. A., & Evers, K. E. (2015). The transtheoretical model and stages of change. In K. Glanz, B. K. Rimer, & K. Viswanath (Eds.), *Health behavior: Theory, research, and practice* (5th ed., pp. 125–148). Jossey-Bass/Wiley.

Rahimi, B., Nadri, H., Lotfnezhad Afshar, H., & Timpka, T. (2018). A systematic review of the technology acceptance model in health informatics. *Applied Clinical Informatics, 9*(3), 604–634. https://doi.org/10.1055/s-0038-1668091

Riley, W. T., Rivera, D. E., Atienza, A. A., Nilsen, W., Allison, S. M., & Mermelstein, R. (2011). Health behavior models in the age of mobile interventions: Are our theories up to the task? *Translational Behavioral Medicine, 1*(1), 53–71. https://doi.org/10.1007/s13142-011-0021-7

Ruggiero, K. J., Bunnell, B. E., Andrews Iii, A. R., Davidson, T. M., Hanson, R. F., Danielson, C. K., Saunders, B. E., Soltis, K., Yarian, C., Chu, B., & Adams, Z. W. (2015). Development and pilot evaluation of a tablet-based application to improve quality of care in child mental health treatment. *JMIR Research Protocols, 4*(4), Article e143. https://doi.org/10.2196/resprot.4416

Ruggiero, K. J., Saunders, B. E., Davidson, T. M., Lewsky Cook, D., & Hanson, R. (2017). Leveraging technology to address the quality chasm in children's evidence-based psychotherapy. *Psychiatric Services, 68*(7), 650–652. https://doi.org/10.1176/appi.ps.201600548

Sachser, C., Berliner, L., Holt, T., Jensen, T. K., Jungbluth, N., Risch, E., Rosner, R., & Goldbeck, L. (2017). International development and psychometric properties of the Child and Adolescent Trauma Screen (CATS). *Journal of Affective Disorders, 210*, 189–195. https://doi.org/10.1016/j.jad.2016.12.040

Schueller, S. M., Armstrong, C. M., Neary, M., & Ciulla, R. P. (2021). An introduction to core competencies for the use of mobile apps. *Cognitive and Behavioral Practice, 29*(1), 69–80. https://doi.org/10.1016/j.cbpra.2020.11.002

Self-Brown, S. R., Osborne, M. C., Rostad, W., & Feil, E. (2017). A technology-mediated approach to the implementation of an evidence-based child maltreatment prevention program. *Child Maltreatment, 22*(4), 344–353. https://doi.org/10.1177/1077559516678482

Silk, J. S., Pramana, G., Sequeira, S. L., Lindhiem, O., Kendall, P. C., Rosen, D., & Parmanto, B. (2020). Using a smartphone app and clinician portal to enhance brief cognitive behavioral therapy for childhood anxiety disorders. *Behavior Therapy, 51*(1), 69–84. https://doi.org/10.1016/j.beth.2019.05.002

Smith, D. L. (2020). *On inhumanity: Dehumanization and how to resist it*. Oxford University Press.

Smith, T. B., & Trimble, J. E. (2016). Matching clients with therapists on the basis of race or ethnicity: A meta-analysis of clients' level of participation. In T. B. Smith & J. E. Trimble (Eds.), *Foundations of multicultural psychology: Research to inform effective practice* (pp. 115–128). American Psychological Association.

Sullivan, A., Forehand, R., Acosta, J., Parent, J., Comer, J. S., Loiselle, R., & Jones, D. J. (2021). COVID-19 and the acceleration of behavioral parent training telehealth: Current status and future directions. *Cognitive and Behavioral Practice, 28*(4), 618–629. https://doi.org/10.1016/j.cbpra.2021.06.012

Titov, N., Dear, B. F., Staples, L. G., Bennett-Levy, J., Klein, B., Rapee, R. M., Shann, C., Richards, D., Andersson, G., Ritterband, L., Purtell, C., Bezuidenhout, G., Johnston, L., & Nielssen, O. B. (2015). MindSpot clinic: An accessible, efficient, and effective online treatment service for anxiety and depression. *Psychiatric Services, 66*(10), 1043–1050. https://doi.org/10.1176/appi.ps.201400477

Torous, J., Stern, A. D. & Bourgeois, F. T. (2022). Regulatory considerations to keep pace with innovation in digital health products. *npj Digital Medicine, 5*(121). https://doi.org/10.1038/s41746-022-00668-9

Vaart, R. van der, & Drossaert, C. (2017). Development of the Digital Health Literacy Instrument: Measuring a broad spectrum of health 1.0 and health 2.0 skills. *Journal of Medical Internet Research, 19*(1), e27. https://doi.org/10.2196/jmir.6709

Vallance, A. K., Hemani, A., Fernandez, V., Livingstone, D., McCusker, K., & Toro-Troconis, M. (2014). Using virtual worlds for role play simulation in child and adolescent psychiatry: An evaluation study. *Psychiatric Bulletin, 38*(5), 204–210. https://doi.org/10.1192/pb.bp.113.044396

Warren, J. C., & Smalley, K. B. (2020). *Using telehealth to meet mental health needs during the COVID-19 crisis*. The Commonwealth Fund. https://www.commonwealthfund.org/blog/2020/using-telehealth-meet-mental-health-needs-during-covid-19-crisis

Weiss, M. D., Baer, S., Allan, B. A., Saran, K., & Schibuk, H. (2011). The screens culture: Impact on ADHD. *Attention Deficit and Hyperactivity Disorders, 3*(4), 327–334. https://doi.org/10.1007/s12402-011-0065-z

Wells, L., & Gowda, A. (2020). A legacy of mistrust: African Americans and the US healthcare system. *Proceedings of UCLA Health*, 24. https://proceedings.med.ucla.edu/wp-content/uploads/2020/06/Wells-A200421LW-rko-Wells-Lindsay-M.D.-BLM-formatted.pdf

Wong Sarver, N., Beidel, D. C., & Spitalnick, J. (2014). The feasibility and acceptability of virtual environments in the treatment of childhood social anxiety disorder. *Journal of Clinical Child and Adolescent Psychology, 43*, 63–73. https://doi.org/10.1080/15374416.2013.843461

# 8

# Appendix: Tools and Resources

**The following materials for your book can be downloaded free of charge once you register on the Hogrefe website:**

Appendix 1: Provider Self-Assessment of Technology Comfort and Attitudes
Appendix 2: Exploring and Identifying a Digital Tool to Integrate Into Child Mental Health Care
Appendix 3: Evaluate the Evidence Base of a Digital Tool for Child Mental Health
Appendix 4: Preparing to Introduce a Digital Tool Into Child Mental Health Care
Appendix 5: Strategies and Tips for Talking to Your Clients About Using Technology as a Part of Care
Appendix 6: Evaluating Client Attitudes About Digital Tools in Child Mental Health Care
Appendix 7: Sample Script for Introducing a Digital Tool Into Child Mental Health Care
Appendix 8: Additional Web-Based Resources

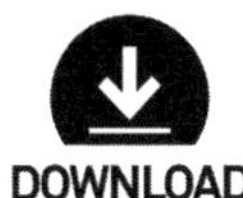


**How to proceed:**

1. Go to www.hgf.io/media and create a user account. If you already have one, please log in.

2. Go to **My supplementary materials** in your account dashboard and enter the code below. You will automatically be redirected to the download area, where you can access and download the supplementary materials.

   **Code: B-3TXK6D**

To make sure you have permanent direct access to all the materials, we recommend that you download them and save them on your computer.

# Appendix 1: Provider Self-Assessment of Technology Comfort and Attitudes

**Instructions:** Before recommending technology use for your clients, it is important that you understand your own comfort with and attitudes toward technology. This assessment is designed to help you evaluate your comfort and identify areas in which additional training or support may be needed. Complete the following questions and consider your readiness for using technology in care.

1. Which of the following technologies do you use at work or in your personal life? (check all that apply)
   - □ Email
   - □ Internet
   - □ Social media (e.g., Twitter, Facebook, Instagram)
   - □ Word processing
   - □ Video conferencing (e.g., Zoom, Skype)
   - □ Mobile/smartphone
   - □ Apps

2. How often do you use a computer?
   a. Daily
   b. 2–6 times a week
   c. Once a week
   d. 2–3 times a month
   e. Once a month
   f. Never

3. How comfortable do you feel using a computer?
   a. Not at all comfortable
   b. A little comfortable
   c. Somewhat comfortable
   d. Very comfortable

4. How comfortable do you feel using the Internet?
   a. Not at all comfortable
   b. A little comfortable
   c. Somewhat comfortable
   d. Very comfortable

5. How comfortable do you feel using mobile apps?
   a. Not at all comfortable
   b. A little comfortable
   c. Somewhat comfortable
   d. Very comfortable

6. I am concerned about using technology with my clients.
   a. Not at all
   b. A little
   c. Somewhat
   d. A lot

7. I believe that technology can improve my clients' experience in therapy.
   a. Not at all
   b. A little
   c. Somewhat
   d. A lot

See p. 71 for instructions on how to obtain the full-sized, printable PDF.

8. I believe that technology will interfere with my relationship with my clients.
    a. Not at all
    b. A little
    c. Somewhat
    d. A lot

9. I believe my clients will be excited to engage with technology as a part of their care.
    a. Not at all
    b. A little
    c. Somewhat
    d. A lot

See p. 71 for instructions on how to obtain the full-sized, printable PDF.

# Appendix 2: Exploring and Identifying a Digital Tool to Integrate Into Child Mental Health Care

**Instructions:** Complete the following questions to practice the process of selecting a digital tool for use with a child or family. We use "mobile app" in our prompts; however, providers can use this worksheet to guide exploration of other digital tools as well.

1. Download a mobile app that you have never used and explore it on your own. What app did you choose and why?
2. What type of client do you think you could use this app with?
   a. Age group?
   b. Gender?
   c. Race/ethnicity?
   d. Sexual orientation?
   e. Presenting problems?
3. How might you use this app in practice with a client?
   a. How would you introduce the app to the family?
   b. How often would you use the app?
   c. Which features would you use?
   d. How would you review completed activities or assessments?

See p. 71 for instructions on how to obtain the full-sized, printable PDF.

# Appendix 3: Evaluate the Evidence Base of a Digital Tool for Child Mental Health

**Instructions:** Complete the following worksheet to determine if a digital tool has adequate evidence to integrate into care. We use "mobile app" in our prompts; however, providers can use this worksheet to guide exploration of other digital tools as well.

1. What evidence-based content (if any) is included in the app (e.g., cognitive restructuring, behavioral activation, breathing techniques, behavioral modification)?
2. What level of evidence is there for this content?
   a. Level 1: Systematic review, meta-analysis, evidence-based guidelines
   b. Level 2: Randomized controlled trial
   c. Level 3: Controlled trial without randomization
   d. Level 4: Nonexperimental study
   e. Level 5: Systematic review of descriptive/qualitative study
   f. Level 6: Descriptive/qualitative study
   g. Level 7: Opinion of authorities, expert panel review
3. Does this existing evidence support use of this content with children or adolescents?
   a. If yes, which age groups?
4. Is there specific evidence for this tool comparing it to the traditional techniques on which the app is based?
5. If yes, what level of evidence?
   a. Level 1: Systematic review, meta-analysis, evidence-based guidelines
   b. Level 2: Randomized controlled trial
   c. Level 3: Controlled trial without randomization
   d. Level 4: Nonexperimental study
   e. Level 5: Systematic review of descriptive/qualitative study
   f. Level 6: Descriptive/qualitative study
   g. Level 7: Opinion of authorities, expert panel review

Now that you have had an opportunity to review the evidence, use your clinical judgment to make decisions about the quality and applicability and tool for your client.

See p. 71 for instructions on how to obtain the full-sized, printable PDF.

# Appendix 4: Preparing to Introduce a Digital Tool Into Child Mental Health Care

**Instructions:** Please answer the questions below to create a comprehensive plan for introducing a digital tool into your child client's care. We use "mobile app" in our prompts; however, providers can use this worksheet to guide exploration of other digital tools as well.

1. How could you introduce the mobile app into a session with your client?
   a. How can the caregiver be included in the discussion?
   b. How do you intend for the child or family to use the app? In session? For homework?
   c. What questions may arise related to privacy or security? Are you prepared to answer these questions?
2. What components of the app could you show the child or caregiver? How can you best demonstrate the potential benefits of using the app to the family?
   a. Would it help to have the child or family practice using the app in session?
   b. Are there components that are not appropriate for this client? If yes, how will you discourage use of those parts?
3. What questions might the child or client have about using the app?
   a. Are there any cultural considerations that might influence the caregiver or child's attitudes toward using the mobile app?
   b. How will you otherwise accomplish the goals of the app if the family refuses, or is unable, to use the tool?

See p. 71 for instructions on how to obtain the full-sized, printable PDF.

# Appendix 5: Strategies and Tips for Talking to Your Clients About Using Technology as a Part of Care

Not all clients are willing or able to use technology as part of their care. It is important to discuss the pros and cons of using technology with your client and to develop a collaborative plan that can be continuously evaluated and refined throughout care. Below are some tips and strategies to consider when talking to your clients about using technology as part of care.

- **Approach the conversation with openness.** Not all clients will feel comfortable engaging with technology as a part of their care. Make sure that you always offer alternatives and are open to adjusting your approach. Client preference is important and should be taken into consideration.
- **Know the advantages and disadvantages.** Make sure you have done your research on the tool or platform that you are recommending. Be ready to answer questions and honestly describe the potential advantages and disadvantages of the digital tool. Be clear about what the tool might offer that other approaches do not and vice versa.
- **Suggest a trial period.** Assess the client's willingness to give it a try. It can often be overwhelming to start something new, so it can be helpful to suggest one feature or aspect of the tool (e.g., relaxation, self-monitoring) for them to focus on. Provide clear expectations.
- **Elicit feedback and be ready to adjust.** Check in with your client weekly about their engagement with and attitudes toward the digital tool. Ask them what they have found to be helpful and what they have not liked. Use this information to guide future recommendations.
- **Include parents or caregivers.** If the youth is using the toolkit independently, ensure that the caregiver has visibility into how their child is interacting with the technology. Make sure you provide a clear rationale for use of the technology and collaboratively set age-appropriate limits on time spent on the device and privacy when using the tool.

See p. 71 for instructions on how to obtain the full-sized, printable PDF.

# Appendix 6: Evaluating Client Attitudes About Digital Tools in Child Mental Health Care

## 1. Assessing Ability and Openness to Mobile App in Care

**Instructions:** Below is a list of questions that you can use to assess the child's or family's ability and openness to use a mobile app in care.

1. Do you own a smartphone or tablet?
   a. If the youth is below the age of 12 assess this with the caregiver first.
   b. If the youth is older than 12 and doesn't have a device, ask caregivers if the child ever uses their device.
   c. If not, discontinue the interview.
2. Do you use your phone or tablet for calls and texting?
   a. This question is designed to assess comfort with technology. If the youth or caregiver does not text, use your clinical judgment to determine whether to proceed with the interview.
3. Do you use your phone for anything else? What kinds of things?
4. Are you familiar with how to download apps from the app store?
   a. If yes, proceed.
   b. If not, use your clinical judgment to determine whether to proceed with introducing the application.
5. Are any of the apps you have downloaded health related (e.g., to count calories, steps, manage sleep)?
   a. If yes, assess how the caregiver or youth uses these apps.
   b. If not, assess their willingness to use an app in treatment or in these ways.
6. Would you be willing to use an app in treatment?
   a. If yes, introduce the app you are interested in and have the caregiver or youth begin the download process.
   b. If not, engage in problem-solving to assess barriers to use (e.g., concerns about cost, privacy, time) and use your clinical judgment about how to proceed.

See p. 71 for instructions on how to obtain the full-sized, printable PDF.

## 2. Strategies and Tips for Challenging and Overcoming Client Hesitation About Technology Use

**Sometimes** clients – either parents or children – are hesitant or reluctant to use technology as a part of their care. Below is a list of strategies and tips for problem-solving. You can use this as a guide in session to inform your conversation and ensure you have enacted a variety of problem-solving skills before deciding not to proceed with the use of technology.

- **Understand what is leading to their hesitancy.** Understanding why your client is reluctant can help determine which strategies will be most effective in overcoming their hesitancy. Common reasons for reluctance include:
  - Lack of comfort or access to technology
  - Concerns about privacy
  - Fear or anxiety of trying something new
  - Resistance to being asked to do something additional
- **Use Socratic questioning and motivational interviewing** to help your client explore their resistance. Rely on your clinical and problem-solving skills just like you would to overcome other therapy-interfering behaviors, like incomplete homework or inconsistent session attendance.
- **Provide a clear rationale for technology use.** Make sure your client understands how you think their engagement with the tool will improve their experience in treatment. Explain why you selected the digital tool, what you hope it will help you track or understand about their experience, and the skills that you think it will help them acquire.
- **Help link technology use to a client-identified goal.** As you explore your client's goals in treatment, think creatively about how the digital tool will help them make and track progress toward these goals. Make sure that you have communicated this clearly with the client.
- **Start small.** Ask your client to give it a try before deciding not to move forward with using a tool. Often, when someone gives something new a try, they learn that it is easier than they previously expected. The same can be true for trying a new technology. Collaboratively pick one feature or activity and have them try it once or twice. In the next session, reassess attitudes.

*Important note:* Not all resistance is bad. If you have made honest attempts to problem-solve and your client remains reluctant, it is okay to move forward without the use of technology. It is important that we meet clients where they are, and client preference is important when considering whether or not to use technology in care.

See p. 71 for instructions on how to obtain the full-sized, printable PDF.

### 3. Strategies and Tips for Improving Client Engagement With Technology

**Consistent** client engagement with digital tools is one of the most common barriers and challenges to using technology in care. Below is a list of strategies and tips for enhancing client engagement. You can use this checklist as a guide before or during sessions to help guide your conversation around technology use.

- **Provide a clear rationale for the incorporation and use of the tool.**
  - What is the intended purpose?
  - Why do you think it will help?

**Collaboratively agree on the tool to be used.**
  - Discuss the pros and cons of different tools.
  - Explore your client's preferences around functionality of the tools.

- **Set clear expectations with the client about use.**
  - How often do you expect them to use the app?
  - Which features of the tool do you expect them to use?
- **Help your client download and set up the tool before they leave session.**
  - Assist in the setup of the app.
  - Practice entering data and navigating the tool.
- **Discuss privacy and security.**
  - Take time in session to explore the tools' privacy settings.
  - When possible, help your client set passwords and enhance privacy settings on their devices.
- **Set up reminders to help prompt engagement.**
  - If the tool has in-app reminders, help your client set them up at a time that is convenient for them.
  - If not, use other reminder systems, like calendar reminders, to prompt engagement.
- **Reinforce engagement in session.**
  - Ask clients about their use of the app between sessions.
  - When possible, access your client's data ahead of session and follow up in session as you would other homework assignments.
  - Provide verbal praise and/or small age-appropriate, physical rewards (e.g., stickers).

See p. 71 for instructions on how to obtain the full-sized, printable PDF.

# Appendix 7: Sample Script for Introducing a Digital Tool Into Child Mental Health Care

This section provides a hypothetical interaction between a therapist and a 14-year-old patient in treatment. The therapist is introducing a mood-monitoring app to be used in conjunction with their weekly face-to-face treatment.

Therapist: Do you have your own smartphone or tablet?
Client: I have a tablet that I use for school.
Therapist: Does the tablet belong to you or the school?
Client: It is mine, but I am only allowed to use it for school if I complete all my homework then my mom lets me go on YouTube.
Therapist: I have an app in mind that I think would be great for us to use while we work together. I am going to bring your mom in to talk about it and see if we can use her phone or your tablet for this. I am going to grab your mom from the waiting room, give me one moment. [The therapist goes to get the client's mom.]
Therapist: Ms. X, I was just talking to your daughter about her tablet. She mentioned that she has one that she uses for school.
Mom: That's right. It is a battle to get her to not use it for other things.
Therapist: I hear that from a lot of parents. Similar to school, I have an app that I think could really help your daughter complete her homework. This app would allow her to keep track of her mood and we could use it in session to track her progress.
Mom: I'm not sure about that. I worry that I won't be able to monitor her.
Therapist: I understand that. What if we looked at the app together and talked about ways that we could monitor her use of it similar to her homework for school.
Client: I don't want her to see what I am doing.
Therapist: I hear that. Does your mom ever check to see if you do your homework without looking at your answers?
Client: Yes.
Therapist: We could come up with something similar to that.
Client: Ok.
Mom: Ok, I am willing to take a look.
Therapist: Would you like me to show you on my phone or would you like to download it on your phone or her tablet, so that you can take a closer look?
Mom: We can use my phone. Wait, how much is this going to cost me?
Therapist: Part of what I like about this tool is that it is free to use. If you could please go to the app store and download [insert name of the app]. While it is downloading, I can tell you more about it.
Mom: Ok. It is downloading.
Therapist: One strategy for improving mood is to increase awareness of how you are feeling overall. We do this by tracking our mood. So to start out, we would like you just to track your mood each day and then we will build on that each week. This app has reminders that prompt you to track your mood and we can set it at a good time for you and a time when you are ok with your daughter using her tablet or your phone.
Mom: That sounds good.
Therapist: Great! If you don't mind, let's get started looking at the app. [Have the caregiver and client create a login and then practice using the app.]
Therapist: How did that feel to use?
Client: I really liked the emojis and it was easy! It took like two seconds.
Mom: I agree that it seems easy.
Therapist: Great! Let's go ahead and set a reminder time and this week I am going to have you give it a try each day and next week we can discuss how it went.

See p. 71 for instructions on how to obtain the full-sized, printable PDF.

# Appendix 8: Additional Web-Based Resources

In addition to the aforementioned resources, we draw the reader's attention to the following websites for more information. Given that these are maintained online, they may not be updated as digital mental health evolves. The list includes sites and resources at the time of our writing that we think may be useful to providers.

**APA Guidelines for the Practice of Telepsychology (2013)**
https://www.apa.org/practice/guidelines/telepsychology

**Child Mind Institute Symptom Checker**
https://childmind.org/symptomchecker/

**Digital Therapeutics Alliance (DTA)**
This has an "Understanding DTx" tab that includes "Foundational Documents" or fact sheets related to the ethics, regulation, and practice of digital therapeutics.
https://dtxalliance.org

**International Society for Research on Internet Interventions**
https://isrii.org

**Limbix: Digital Therapeutics for Adolescent Mental Health**
https://www.limbix.com

**Mental Health Innovation Network**
https://www.mhinnovation.net

**National Health Service Apps Library**
https://digital.nhs.uk/services/nhs-apps-library

**One Mind PsyberGuide: Apps and Digital Health Resources Reviewed by Experts**
https://onemindpsyberguide.org

**ORCHA**
https://orchahealth.com/services/digital-health-libraries/

**Our Mobile Health**
https://www.ourmobilehealth.com

**Rural Health Information Hub**
https://www.ruralhealthinfo.org/toolkits/telehealth/2/specific-populations/children

**Sesame Street Workshop Apps and Ebooks**
See Resources tab.
https://www.sesamestreet.org/apps

**Veterans Administration Mobile App Store**
https://mobile.va.gov/appstore

See p. 71 for instructions on how to obtain the full-sized, printable PDF.